BLUEPRINTS
Q&A Step 3 Surgery

Second Edition

BLUEPRINTS
Q&A Step 3 Surgery

Second Edition

Edward W. Nelson, MD
Professor of Surgery
University of Utah
Attending Surgeon
University of Utah Medical Center
Salt Lake City, Utah

Series Editor:

Michael S. Clement, MD, FAAP
Mountain Park Health Center
Clinical Lecturer in Family and Community Medicine
University of Arizona College of Medicine
Consultant, Arizona Department of Health Services
Phoenix, Arizona

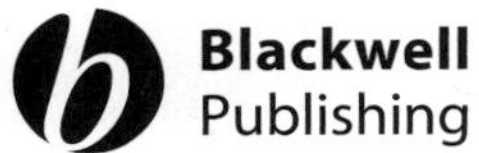

Blackwell Publishing, Inc., 350 Main Street, Malden, Massachusetts 02148-5018, USA
Blackwell Publishing Ltd, 9600 Garsington Road, Oxford OX4 2DQ, UK
Blackwell Publishing Asia Pty Ltd, 550 Swanston Street, Carlton, Victoria 3053, Australia

04 05 06 07 5 4 3 2 1

ISBN: 1-4051-0398-1

Library of Congress Cataloging-in-Publication Data

Blueprints Q&A step 3. Surgery / [edited by] Edward W. Nelson.—2nd ed.
p. ; cm.
Includes index.
ISBN 1-4051-0398-1 (pbk.)
1. Surgery—Examinations, questions, etc. 2. Physicians—Licenses—United States—Examinations—Study guides.
[DNLM: 1. Surgery—Examination Questions. 2. Surgical Procedures, Operative—Examination Questions. WO 18.2 B6582 2005]
I. Title: Blueprints Q and A step three. Surgery. II. Title: Surgery.
III. Nelson, Edward W.
RD37.2.B582 2005
617'. 0076—dc22

2004013548

A catalogue record for this title is available from the British Library.

Acquisitions: Nancy Anastasi Duffy
Development: Kate Heinle
Production: Jennifer Kowalewski
Cover design: Hannus Design Associates
Interior design: Mary McKeon
Typesetter: TechBooks, in New Delhi, India
Printed and bound by Capital City Press, in Berlin, VT

For further information on Blackwell Publishing, visit our website:
www.blackwellmedstudent.com

Notice: The indications and dosages of all drugs in this book have been recommended in the medical literature and conform to the practices of the general community. The medications described do not necessarily have specific approval by the Food and Drug Administration for use in the diseases and dosages for which they are recommended. The package insert for each drug should be consulted for use and dosage as approved by the FDA. Because standards for usage change, it is advisable to keep abreast of revised recommendations, particularly those concerning new drugs.

The publisher's policy is to use permanent paper from mills that operate a sustainable forestry policy, and which has been manufactured from pulp processed using acid-free and elementary chlorine-free practices. Furthermore, the publisher ensures that the text paper and cover board used have met acceptable environmental accreditation standards.

Contents

Contributors

Rafe C. Connors, MD
Resident, Department of General Surgery
University of Utah School of Medicine
Salt Lake City, Utah

Stephen J. Fenton, MD
Resident, Department of General Surgery
University of Utah School of Medicine
Salt Lake City, Utah

Faculty Reviewers

Courtney L. Scaife, MD
Assistant Professor of Surgery
University of Utah School of Medicine
Salt Lake City, Utah

Michelle T. Mueller, MD
Assistant Professor of Surgery
University of Utah School of Medicine
Salt Lake City, Utah

Reviewers

Jonathan Gottlieb, MD
Resident, Orthopedic Surgery
University of Miami
Miami, Florida

Adam D. Fox, DPM, DO
Resident, Department of Surgery
Christiana Care Health System
Newark, Delaware

Marineh Yaguban, MD
Resident, General Surgery
Mayo Clinic
Rochester, Minnesota

Preface

Thank you! We know that you, our customers, have successfully used the first edition of the *Blueprints Q&A* series to study for Boards and shelf exams. We also learned that those of you in physician assistant, nurse practitioner, and osteopath programs have found the series helpful to review for boards and rotation exams.

At Blackwell, we think of our customers as our secret weapon. For every book Blackwell publishes, we rely heavily on the opinions of our customers, and we credit much of our success to the feedback we get from you. Your comments, suggestions—even complaints—help determine everything from content to features to the design of our books. The second edition of the *Blueprints Q&A* series is an excellent example of how much influence your feedback truly has:

- You asked for more questions per book, so the questions have doubled (200 per book!).
- You wanted questions that better reflect the current format of the Boards, so all questions have been updated to match the current USMLE format for Step 3.
- You liked the detailed explanations for every answer—right or wrong—so we made sure that complete correct and incorrect answers were provided for each question.
- You needed a smaller trim size for easier portability, and now you have it. This edition is small enough to fit in a white coat pocket.
- You were looking for an easier way to test yourself, and we redesigned this edition to do just that. Answer keys and tabbed sections make for easier navigation between questions and answers.
- You wanted an index for easy reference, and you got it (along with abbreviations and normal lab values).

We hope you like this new edition of the *Blueprints Q&A* series as much as we do. And keep your suggestions and ideas coming! Please send any comments you may have about this book, or any book in the *Blueprints* series, to *blue@bos.blackwellpublishing.com*.

The Publisher
Blackwell Publishing

Acknowledgments

The goal of this review was to provide the appropriate scope and quality of information to adequately prepare students for the surgical portions of the USMLE Step 3 exam. The extent to which that goal has been accomplished is entirely attributable to the efforts of my resident authors, Rafe and Steve, and to our faculty reviewers, Michelle and Courtney. Most importantly, we are all indebted to Mary Mone, our collaborator, counsel, and conscience throughout.

—Edward W. Nelson

Abbreviations

μU	micro international unit
5-HIAA	5-hydroxyindoleacetic acid
AAA	abdominal aortic aneurysm
ABC	airway, breathing, circulation
ABG	arterial blood gas
ABI	ankle brachial index
ACAS	Asymptomatic Carotid Atherosclerosis Study
ACOSOG	American College of Surgeons Oncology Group
ACS	abdominal compartment syndrome
ACTH	adrenocorticotropic hormone
ADH	antidiuretic hormone
AFP	alpha fetoprotein
AHA	autoimmune hemolytic anemia
ALS	amyotrophic lateral sclerosis
ALT	alanine aminotransferase
APUD	amine precursor uptake and decarboxylation
ARDS	acute respiratory distress syndrome
AST	aspartate aminotransferase
ATN	acute tubular necrosis
AV	arteriovenous
AV	atrioventricular
AVM	arteriovenous malformation
BE	base excess
BMP	basic metabolic panel
BP	blood pressure
BPH	benign prostatic hypertrophy
BRCA	breast cancer gene 1 or 2
BUN	blood urea nitrogen
BW	body weight
C	Celsius; centigrade
C	cervical
Ca	calcium
CABG	coronary artery bypass graft
cAMP	cyclic adenosine monophosphate
CBC	complete blood count
cc	cubic centimeter
CCU	coronary care unit
CEA	carcinoembryonic antigen
CI	cardiac index
Cl	chloride
cm	centimeter
CML	chronic myelogenous leukemia
CNS	central nervous system
CO	cardiac output
CO_2	carbon dioxide
CPAP	continuous positive airway pressure
CPK-MB	creatinine phosphokinase-myocardial
CPM	central pontine myelinolysis
CT	cardiothoracic
CT	computed tomography
CTA	computed tomography angiography
CVA	cerebral vascular accident
CVP	central venous pressure
CXR	chest x-ray
d	day
DA	duodenal atresia
DCIS	ductal carcinoma in situ
DHEA	dehydroepiandrosterone
DI	diabetes insipidus
DKA	diabetic ketoacidois
dL	deciliter
DVT	deep vein thrombosis
ECF	extracellular fluid
ECF	enterocutaneous fistula
ECG	electrocardiogram
ECMO	extracorporeal membrane oxygenation
ED	emergency department
EGD	esophagogastroduodenoscopy
EMS	emergency medical service
ER	emergency room
ERCP	endoscopic retrograde cholangiopancreatography
ERU	endorectal ultrasound
F	Fahrenheit
FFP	fresh frozen plasma
FiO_2	fraction of inspired oxygen

FNA fine-needle aspiration
g gram
G gravida
GCS Glasgow Coma Scale
GE gastroesophageal
GERD gastroesophageal reflux disease
GI gastrointestinal
H_2 histamine 2 receptor
HCC hepatocellular carcinoma
hCG human chorionic gonadotropin
HCO_3 bicarbonate
HCT hematocrit
HER-2 human epidermal growth factor receptor-2
HIDA hydroxy iminodiacetic acid
HNPCC hereditary nonpolyposis colon cancer
HPV human papillomavirus
HR heart rate
HVA homovanillic acid
I^{131} iodine-131
IAP intra-abdominal pressure
IBD inflammatory bowel disease
ICP intracranial pressure
ICU intensive care unit
IgG immunoglobulin G
IL interleukin
INR international ratio
ITP idiopathic thrombocytopenic purpura
IUD intra-uterine device
IV intravenous
IVC inferior vena cava
IVIG intravenous immunoglobulin
IVP intravenous pyelogram
K potassium
kcal kilocalorie
kg kilogram
KUB kidney, ureter, bladder
L lumbar
L liter
LAD left anterior descending
lb pound
LCIS lobular carcinoma in situ
LDH lactic dehydrogenase
LES lower esophageal sphincter
LUQ left upper quadrant
LVAD left ventricular assist device
m meter
MALT mucosa-associated lymphoid tissue lymphoma
MAST military anti-shock trousers
MEN multiple endocrine neoplasia
mEq milliequivalent
mg milligram
Mg magnesium
mg/dL milligram per deciliter
MI myocardial infarction
MIBG meta-iodobenzylguanidine
min minute
mIU milli-international unit
mm millimeter
mm Hg millimeters of mercury
mmol millimole
MRI magnetic resonance imaging
MTC medullary thyroid cancer
Na sodium
$NaHCO_3$ sodium bicarbonate
NASCET North American Symptomatic Carotid Endarterectomy Trial
NEC necrotizing enterocolitis
NG nasogastric
ng nanogram
NGT nasogastric tube
NJ nasojejeunal
NPO nothing by mouth
NS normal saline
NSABP National Surgical Adjuvant Bowel and Breast Project
NSAID nonsteroidal anti-inflammatory drug
O_2 oxygen
1,25 $(OH)_2D_3$ 1,25-dihydroxyvitamin D_3
OPSI overwhelming post-splenectomy infection
OR operating room
P para; parity
PA posterior-anterior
PA pulmonary artery
PCO_2 arterial carbon dioxide pressure
PO_2 arterial oxygen pressure
PCWP pulmonary capillary wedge pressure
PE pulmonary embolism
PEEP positive end expiratory pressure
pH hydrogen ion concentration
PID pelvic inflammatory disease
PIP peak inspiratory pressure
Plt platelet
PMN polymorphonuclear
PO_4 phosphate
PP pancreatic polypeptide
PSA prostate-specific antigen
PSC primary sclerosing cholangitis
PT prothrombin time
PTCH percutaneous transhepatic cholangiography
PTH parathyroid hormone

PTHC	percutaneous transhepatic cholangiography
PTT	partial thromboplastin time
PTU	propylthiouracil
PVC	polyvinyl chloride
PVD	peripheral vascular disease
qid	four times a day
RA	room air
RA	rheumatoid arthritis
RB	retinoblastoma
RBC	red blood cell
RCC	renal cell carcinoma
REE	resting energy expenditure
RET	REarranged during Transfection oncogene
RL	ringer's lactate
RR	respiratory rate
RUQ	right upper quadrant
RVAD	right ventricular assist device
s	second
S	sacral
SaO_2	arterial oxygen saturation
SBFT	small bowel follow-through
SBO	small bowel obstruction
SCC	squamous cell carcinoma
SG	Swan-Ganz
SIADH	syndrome of inappropriate antidiuretic hormone
SICU	surgical intensive care unit
SRU	solitary rectal ulcer
SSI	surgical skin infection
STD	sexually transmitted disease
SVR	systemic vascular resistance
T	thoracic
T	temperature
T_3	tri-iodothyronine
T_4	thyroxine
TBSA	total body surface area
TBW	total body water
TEE	transesophageal echocardiogram
TIA	transient ischemic attack
TIPSS	transjugular intrahepatic portosystemic shunt
TNF	tumor necrosis factor
TOA	tubo-ovarian abscess
TPN	total parenteral nutrition
TSH	thyroid-stimulating hormone
TURBT	transurethral resection of bladder tumor
TURP	transurethral resection of the prostate
U/L	international units per liter
UA	urinalysis
UC	ulcerative colitis
US	ultrasound
UTI	urinary tract infection
V_E	minute ventilation
VIP	vasoactive intestinal peptide
VMA	vanillylmandelic acid
V_T	tidal volume
WBC	white blood cell

Normal Ranges of Laboratory Values

Chemistry

Alanine aminotransferase (ALT)	Male: 13–72 U/L, Female: 9–52 U/L
Alkaline phosphatase	38–126 U/L
Amylase	30–110 U/L
Aspartate aminotransferase (AST)	Male: 15–59 U/L, Female: 14–50
Bicarbonate (HCO_3^-)	19–25 mmol/L
Bilirubin total	0.2–1.3 mg/dL
Bilirubin direct	0.0–0.3 mg/dL
Calcium	8.4–10.2 mg/dL
Carbon dioxide	22–29 mmol/L
Chloride (Cl^-)	98–107 mmol/L
Creatinine	Male: 0.8–1.5 mg/dL, Female: 0.7–1.2 mg/dL
Glucose	64–128 mg/dL
Lactate	0.7–2.1 mmol/L
Lactate dehydrogenase (LDH)	300–600 U/L
Magnesium (Mg^{2+})	1.6–2.3 mg/dL
Osmolality	280–303 mOsm/kg
Potassium (K^+)	3.3–5.0 mmol/L
Phosphorus (inorganic)	2.4–4.3 mg/dL
Sodium (Na^+)	136–144 mmol/L
Urea nitrogen (BUN)	Male: 9–22 mg/dL, Female: 6–22

Hematologic

Hematocrit	Male: 40.8–51.9%, Female: 34.3–46.6%
Hemoglobin	Male: 14.6–17.8 g/dL, Female: 12.1–15.9 g/dL
Leukocyte count	3200–10,600/mm^3
Partial thromboplastin time	26–37 s
Platelet count	177,000–406,000 K/μL
Prothrombin time	12–15.5 s

Reproduced by permission of Associated Regional and University Pathologists (ARUP) Laboratories, Salt Lake City, Utah.

Block

ONE

Questions

Setting 1: Community-Based Health Center

You work at a community-based health facility where patients seeking both routine and urgent care are encountered. Many patients are members of low-income groups; many are ethnic minorities. Several industrial parks and local businesses send their employees to the health center for treatment of on-the-job injuries and employee health screening. There is a facility that provides x-ray films, but CT and MRI scans must be arranged at other facilities. Laboratory services are available.

The next three questions (items 1–3) correspond to the following vignette.

A 33-year-old female is seen at your clinic complaining of a 2-month history of diarrhea and intermittent abdominal pain. Prior to her current problem, she was healthy without any medications or prior surgeries. Review of symptoms reveals a recent 25-pound weight loss and recurrent mouth sores. On physical exam, the patient is cachectic with a soft, nontender abdomen. A colonoscopy with biopsy is scheduled for the next day.

1. Which of the following is characteristic of this clinical setting?

  A. Sclerosing cholangitis
  B. Rectal involvement
  C. Treatment via ileoanal pouch procedure
  D. Linear ulcers
  E. Rectal bleeding

2. Your suspicion is confirmed with the biopsies obtained, and medical management is initiated. One year later, the patient is admitted to the hospital due to nausea and vomiting with abdominal pain and distention. An abdominal CT is obtained (Figure 2A). Treatment with bowel rest, nasogastric decompression, and IV fluids is instituted. What is the most likely diagnosis?

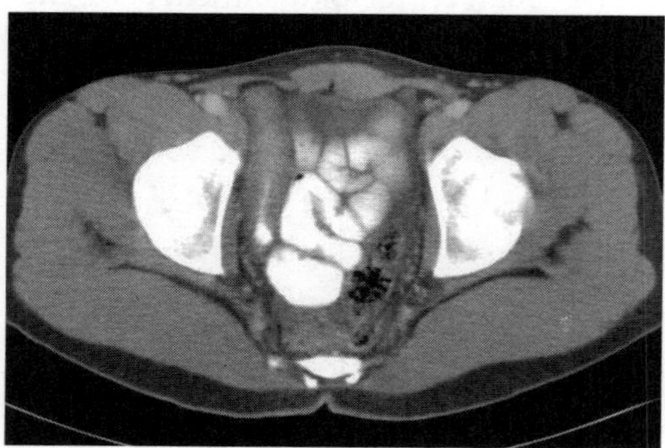

Figure 2A • Image courtesy of the University of Utah School of Medicine, Salt Lake City, Utah.

  A. Adhesions
  B. Stricture
  C. Volvulus
  D. Femoral hernia
  E. Pelvic abscess

3. Which of the following is an extra-intestinal manifestation of IBD?

  A. Abdominal pain
  B. Risk of carcinoma
  C. Thickened bowel wall
  D. Sclerosing cholangitis
  E. Lymphoid aggregation

End of set

The next two questions (items 4 and 5) correspond to the following vignette.

A 50-year-old male with known ulcerative colitis visits your clinic. The patient complains of abdominal pain, pruritus, malaise, fever, and a recent 15-pound weight loss. History includes a total colectomy more than 10 years ago. On physical exam, the patient has mild scleral icterus and is tender in the right upper quadrant.

4. What is the most appropriate next step in this patient's management?

- **A.** Exploratory laparotomy
- **B.** CT scan of abdomen
- **C.** ERCP
- **D.** MRI of the abdomen
- **E.** Colonoscopy

5. As this disease progresses, it will most likely result in the need for which surgery?

- **A.** Laparoscopic cholecystectomy
- **B.** Liver transplant
- **C.** Choledochojejunostomy
- **D.** Open cholecystectomy
- **E.** Whipple procedure

End of set

The next two questions (items 6 and 7) correspond to the following vignette.

A 67-year-old male comes to your clinic complaining of a 2-day history of persistent nausea and vomiting, without relief from use of over-the-counter medications. The last time this patient saw a doctor was 2 years ago. The patient reports to you that he has not had any previous medical problems, takes no medications, and has had a remote appendectomy. On physical exam, the patient appears acutely ill and is tachycardic, with a benign abdominal exam. The following labs are obtained: Na, 147 mmol/L; K, 4 mmol/L; Cl, 110 mmol/L; BUN, 25 mg/dL; Cr, 1.0 mg/dL; glucose, 120 mg/dL; Ca, 13.5 mg/dL.

6. What is the most appropriate first step in management of this patient?

- **A.** PTH levels
- **B.** Furosemide administration
- **C.** Sestamibi scan
- **D.** IV hydration
- **E.** Plicamycin

7. This patient's disorder will cause which of the following lab values?

- **A.** Increased PTH, decreased serum calcium, increased serum phosphate
- **B.** Increased PTH, increased serum calcium, decreased serum phosphate
- **C.** Decreased PTH, increased serum calcium, increased serum phosphate
- **D.** Decreased PTH, decreased serum calcium, increased serum phosphate
- **E.** Normal PTH, normal serum calcium, normal serum phosphate

End of set

The next two questions (items 8 and 9) correspond to the following vignette.

A 63-year-old male with a 55-pack-per-year history of smoking and a 35-pound weight loss over the last 4 months presents to your community-based health center with the complaint of blood in his urine for the last 3 weeks. You obtain a urinalysis and confirm the presence of hematuria. You are concerned for the possibility of bladder cancer.

8. Which of the following is the most accurate means of confirming your diagnosis?

A. Urine culture
B. Intravenous pyelogram
C. Cystoscopy with directed and random biopsies
D. Bladder washings for cytology
E. MRI of the abdomen and pelvis

9. The patient is diagnosed with a transitional cell cancer of the bladder. A transurethral resection of the bladder tumor (TURBT) is performed through the cystoscope. The tumor is found to be superficial on pathology, with no evidence of invasive or metastatic disease. Regarding bladder cancer, what can generally be stated about treatment, cell type, or the degree of invasiveness?

A. Most bladder tumors are transitional cell and superficial in depth.
B. Most bladder tumors are transitional cell and invasive beyond the lamina propria.
C. Most bladder tumors are metastatic when diagnosed.
D. Most bladder tumors are high grade, aneuploid when diagnosed.
E. Most bladder tumors require chemotherapy.

End of set

The next three questions (items 10–12) correspond to the following vignette.

A 67-year-old male presents to your community-based health center with a history of weight loss, chronic cough, and hemoptysis. The patient has a 65-pack-per-year smoking history. You obtain a chest x-ray, which shows a mass near the hilum of the lung. A CT scan (Figure 10) confirms the presence of a centrally located 3 cm mass (indicated by arrow).

10. What is the most appropriate next step in management?

A. Repeat the CT scan in 6 months to look for advancement of the tumor
B. CT-guided biopsy of the mass
C. Bronchoscopy with transbronchial biopsy
D. Mediastinoscopy
E. Thoracoscopy with biopsy

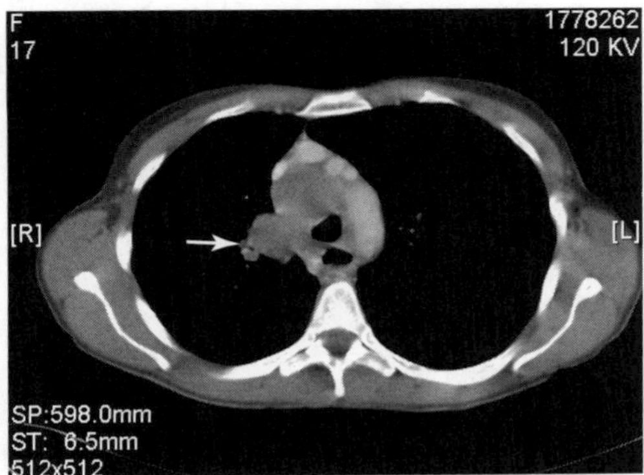

Figure 10 • Image courtesy of the University of Utah School of Medicine, Salt Lake City, Utah.

11. When you receive the pathology report of your biopsy 5 days later, you determine the mass to be unresectable based solely on the biopsy results. Which of the following tumor histologies has the most aggressive natural history?

A. Squamous cell carcinoma
B. Adenocarcinoma
C. Small cell carcinoma
D. Large cell carcinoma
E. Hodgkin's disease

12. If the pathology report on this patient showed the tumor to be a squamous cell carcinoma, which paraneoplastic syndrome would he be at most risk for developing?

A. SIADH
B. Eaton-Lambert syndrome
C. PTH-like peptide syndrome
D. Cushing's syndrome
E. Ectopic acromegaly

End of set

The next two questions (items 13 and 14) correspond to the following vignette.

You see a 64-year-old homeless Caucasian male in the outreach clinic who is complaining of abdominal distention. The patient was diagnosed with cirrhosis of the liver secondary to hepatitis C infection more than 10 years ago. The patient has not seen a physician in more than 5 years.

13. Which of the following is used in determining this patient's Child's classification?

- **A.** Age
- **B.** History of smoking
- **C.** Encephalopathy
- **D.** Hepatocellular enzyme elevation (ALT, AST)
- **E.** PTT

14. You determine that the patient fits the definition of Child's class B. The patient also gives a history concerning for diabetes, coronary artery disease, and a 45-pack-per-year history of smoking. What is the best option for intervention for this patient with esophageal varices?

- **A.** Mesocaval shunt "H" graft
- **B.** Transjugular intrahepatic portosystemic shunt
- **C.** Warren distal splenorenal shunt
- **D.** End-to-side portal caval shunt
- **E.** Emergent liver transplant

End of set

---

15. A 6-week-old male infant is brought to your clinic because of a 2-week history of emesis. The mother describes the emesis as nonbilious and reports it has become projectile over the last 48 hours. On physical exam, the infant's abdomen is soft and a palpable mass is detected in the right upper quadrant. A contrast study is obtained (Figures 15A and 15B). What is this child's most likely diagnosis?

- **A.** Duodenal atresia
- **B.** Cholangiocarcinoma
- **C.** Hirschsprung disease
- **D.** Hypertrophic pyloric stenosis
- **E.** Intestinal malrotation

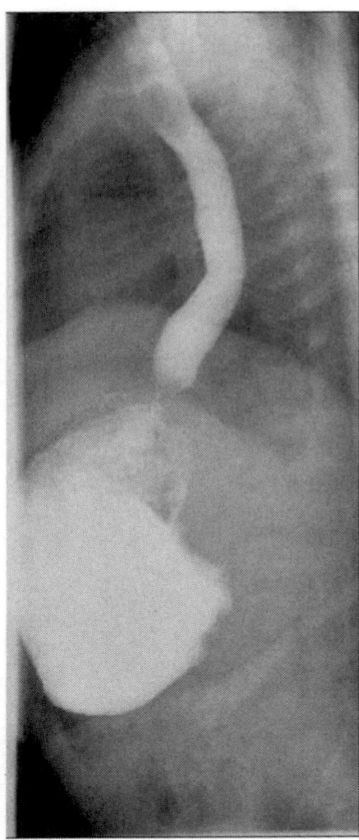

Figure 15A • Image courtesy of the University of Utah School of Medicine, Salt Lake City, Utah.

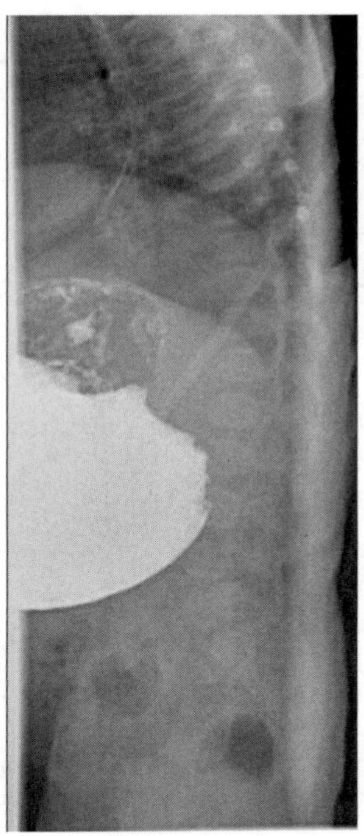

Figure 15B • Image courtesy of the University of Utah School of Medicine, Salt Lake City, Utah.

16. A 60-year-old male comes to your clinic with a large mass in his groin that he believes is a hernia. The patient has had this mass for the last 6 months, and it had been easily reducible until this morning. The mass has become increasingly more painful, and the patient is experiencing nausea and vomiting. On exam, the mass is tender to palpation and the hernia appears incarcerated. After giving the patient some midazolam and morphine sulfate in the clinic procedure room, you are still unable to reduce the hernia. What is the next step in management of this patient?

A. Have the patient return in 12 hours for reevaluation
B. Ultrasound of the mass
C. CT scan of the abdomen and pelvis
D. Upper GI imaging with small bowel follow-through
E. Emergency surgery

The next two questions (items 17 and 18) correspond to the following vignette.

A 72-year-old male comes to your clinic complaining of a 2-day history of urinary hesitancy, frequent urination, and discomfort upon urinating. A urinalysis demonstrates bacteria, more than 75 WBC, and the presence of leukocyte esterase and nitrites. The patient has non-insulin-dependent diabetes and suffers from arthritis. Currently the patient is not taking any medications. Surgical history includes an appendectomy, cholecystectomy, and cataract surgery. Vital signs are normal. On physical exam, the patient is thin, but otherwise well developed. There is no urethral discharge, and his testicles are nontender to examination. A rectal exam reveals a large, smooth prostate. The remainder of his exam is unremarkable.

17. What is the most likely etiology of these symptoms?

A. Gonorrhea
B. Prostate cancer
C. Kidney stone
D. Hydronephrosis
E. Bladder outlet obstruction
F. Rectal cancer

18. After initial medical management, the patient returns to your clinic 2 months later to report that the symptoms initially improved, but later returned and recently have become significantly worse. You recommend a transurethral resection of the prostate. What should you tell the patient regarding risks if the proposed procedure reveals prostatic cancer?

A. Prostate cancer is rarely fatal
B. Caucasians are the most likely to develop cancer
C. Risk factors include a high-fat diet and tobacco consumption
D. Prostate cancers are universally indolent
E. The majority of patients have locally or metastatic disease when diagnosed

End of set

---

19. An 18-month-old male is referred to your clinic by his pediatrician for evaluation of right cryptorchidism. On exam, you are unable to palpate his right testicle and note that his left testicle had descended properly into the scrotum. What is the most appropriate management of this child's cryptorchidism?

A. Ultrasound
B. CT scan of the abdomen and pelvis
C. Orchiectomy
D. Surgical exploration and scrotal placement of the testicle
E. Wait until age 4 before operating to allow time for descent of the testicle

The next two questions (items 20 and 21) correspond to the following vignette.

A 38-year-old African American patient with diabetes comes to your outreach clinic complaining of rectal pain and fevers up to 103.1°F. On exam the patient reports that the onset of pain was approximately 5 days ago; it has gotten progressively worse since that time. Fevers started 2 days ago and subside somewhat with acetaminophen administration, but they return as the medication wears off. The only abnormal lab is the WBC, which is 14,800. You perform a rectal exam and find a fluctuant mass on the anterior rectal wall.

20. What is the best initial treatment for this patient's problem?

- **A.** Admission and IV antibiotics
- **B.** Referral to radiology for needle drainage
- **C.** Localization via CT
- **D.** Evaluation via endorectal ultrasound (ERU)
- **E.** Surgical drainage

21. Which of the following is a relatively common sequela of this condition?

- **A.** Anal incontinence
- **B.** Colovesical fistula
- **C.** Anal stricture
- **D.** Fistula in ano
- **E.** Anal fissure

End of set

---

22. A 42-year-old female visits your clinic for her annual mammogram and breast exam. Upon examination, both her breasts appear normal and there are no palpable masses. The radiology report for the mammogram states there is an area concerning for ductal carcinoma in situ (DCIS). DCIS is a precursor lesion to invasive ductal carcinoma and is treated with surgical resection. Which of the following statements is true of DCIS?

- **A.** DCIS is usually found on physical exam.
- **B.** Microcalcifications are usually seen on mammogram in DCIS.
- **C.** Lumpectomy with axillary dissection is the surgery of choice.
- **D.** Radiation therapy has no role in the treatment of DCIS.
- **E.** There is a high risk of lymph node involvement in DCIS.

The next two questions (items 23 and 24) correspond to the following vignette.

A 29-year-old Hispanic male with a 3-week history of vague abdominal pain is referred to your clinic. The patient has been living in the United States for the past 4 months, and he has no prior history of medical illness or surgery. In addition to the pain, the patient complains of some fever and chills, and he has no desire to eat. Vital signs are as follows: T 38.1°C, HR 85, BP 132/65, RR 12, SaO_2 95% on room air. On your exam, the patient is ill appearing, and has fullness in the right upper quadrant associated with pain upon palpation. You observe the following CT scan (Figure 23A).

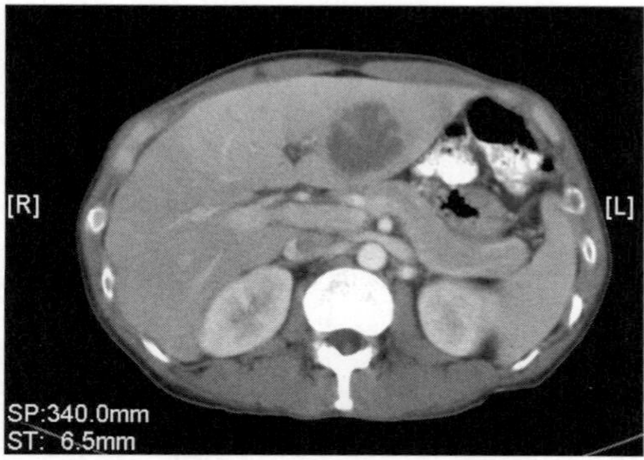

Figure 23A • Image courtesy of the University of Utah School of Medicine, Salt Lake City, Utah.

23. Which of the following tests is most likely to aid in the diagnosis of this patient's disease?

- **A.** Liver function test
- **B.** Indirect hemagglutination titer
- **C.** Complete blood count
- **D.** Indirect Coombs' test
- **E.** Chemistry panel

24. What is the most appropriate initial management of this disease?

- **A.** Oral metronidazole with percutaneous drainage
- **B.** Operative drainage
- **C.** Oral metronidazole
- **D.** IV gentamicin/ampicillin/metronidazole with percutaneous drainage
- **E.** IV gentamicin/ampicillin/metronidazole

End of set

The next three questions (items 25–27) correspond to the following vignette.

A 37-year-old female is referred to clinic due to a hepatic mass found on CT scan. The patient denies current right upper quadrant pain and is otherwise healthy. A thorough investigation for cancer by her primary care physician revealed nothing. Patient history does not include any prior abdominal surgery or recent travel outside the United States, but she is allergic to penicillin and takes NSAIDs for occasional headaches. The patient is afebrile and hemodynamically stable, and her labs are within normal limits. You observe the following CT scan (Figure 25A).

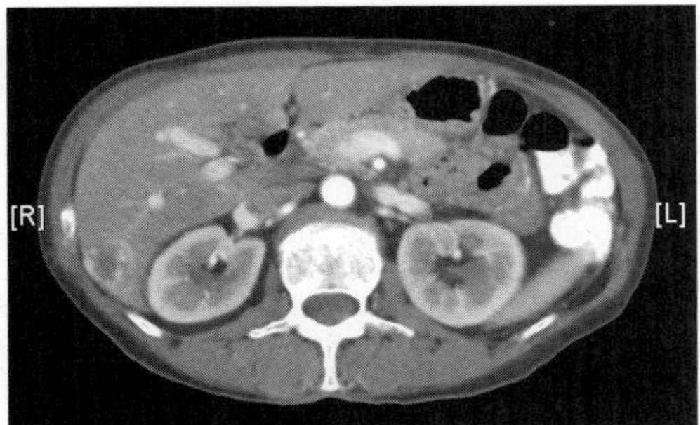

Figure 25A • Image courtesy of the University of Utah School of Medicine, Salt Lake City, Utah.

25. What is the most likely diagnosis?

- **A.** Hepatic hemangioma
- **B.** Hamartoma
- **C.** Hepatocellular carcinoma
- **D.** Bacterial abscess
- **E.** Hydatid cyst

26. Which of the following is the best initial treatment?

- **A.** Hepatic wedge resection
- **B.** Percutaneous drainage
- **C.** Hepatic lobectomy
- **D.** Observation
- **E.** Sclerotherapy

27. Which of the following is the most common worldwide cause of hepatocellular carcinoma?

- **A.** Polyvinyl chloride
- **B.** Hepatitis B
- **C.** Hepatitis A
- **D.** Cirrhosis
- **E.** Aflatoxins

End of set

The next three questions (items 28–30) correspond to the following vignette.

A 21-year-old male presents to the emergency department with a 15-hour history of abdominal pain associated with vomiting and a fever. The pain localizes to the right lower quadrant and the WBC count approaches 13,000. The patient undergoes a laparoscopic appendectomy without incident and is discharged from the hospital the next day. The appendectomy pathology report shows a 3 cm small cell tumor at the base of the appendix.

28. What is the correct treatment at this point?

- **A.** Right hemicolectomy
- **B.** Radiation therapy
- **C.** Hepatic wedge resection
- **D.** Observation alone
- **E.** Trastuzumab

29. At follow-up in your clinic 1 week after hospital discharge, the patient describes a 4-month history of weight loss and fatigue. The patient also states that he has had loose, watery stools with a decreased appetite. On exam he appears somewhat flushed, and you appreciate end expiratory wheezes throughout both lung fields. The history and findings are most consistent with which tumor?

- **A.** Adenocarcinoma
- **B.** Insulinoma
- **C.** Lymphoma
- **D.** Gastrinoma
- **E.** Carcinoid

30. Which of the following tests is most appropriate in confirming the diagnosis?

- **A.** Serum gastrin
- **B.** Serum protein C
- **C.** Colonoscopy
- **D.** Urinary 5-hydroxyindoleacetic acid (5-HIAA)
- **E.** Urinary metanephrine

End of set

The next two questions (items 31 and 32) correspond to the following vignette.

A 30-year-old male visits your clinic with complaints of drainage around his anus. Perianal pain began 1 week ago and increased until yesterday when it acutely improved, but the patient began noticing drainage from this area. The patient has become constipated due to his reluctance to have a bowel movement. Otherwise the patient is healthy, denies allergies, and is not taking any medication. Examination reveals a slightly erythematous area that appears to have spontaneously drained purulent material and has left an open cavity that is freely draining. It is located just lateral to the anus.

31. What is the best next step in this patient's management?

- **A.** Pack with wet-to-dry saline-soaked gauze
- **B.** Rectal irrigations with saline-mixed antibiotics
- **C.** IV antibiotics
- **D.** Incision and drainage
- **E.** Warm sitz baths

32. The dentate line is an important surgical landmark in the anus. Which of the following statements best describes this landmark and its significance?

- **A.** Below the dentate line the innervation is primarily autonomic.
- **B.** Stratified squamous epithelium is found above the dentate line, whereas columnar epithelium is found below it.
- **C.** The blood supply, both above and below the dentate line, is derived from the superior rectal artery.
- **D.** The dentate line defines the level above which transanal excisions are impossible.
- **E.** There is embryologic differentiation between endoderm and ectoderm.
- **F.** Malignant cells from above the dentate line will drain to the inguinal lymph nodes.

End of set

The next two questions (items 33 and 34) correspond to the following vignette.

A distraught young mother brings her 10-month-old male infant to your clinic. The mother tells you that the child began acting differently yesterday afternoon, by not being as playful as usual and not wanting to eat. This behavior was followed by vomiting green fluid. According to the mother, the child has become increasingly lethargic, which prompted her to bring him in. On physical exam, the child appears ill and is lying still, the abdomen is distended and diffusely tender, and no peritoneal signs are present. Abdominal films are obtained and are consistent with an obstructive process.

33. What is the next step in management of this patient?

- **A.** Upper GI imaging with small bowel follow-through
- **B.** Esophagogastroduodenoscopy
- **C.** Barium enema
- **D.** Emergent exploratory laparotomy
- **E.** Colonoscopy

34. Imaging is performed, and results are consistent with malrotation and midgut volvulus. What is the most appropriate next step?

- **A.** Endoscopy
- **B.** IV resuscitation and observation
- **C.** Gastrografin enema
- **D.** Air-contrast enema
- **E.** Exploratory laparotomy

End of set

---

35. A 55-year-old female presents to your outreach clinic complaining of an itchy right breast. The patient tells you that she has noticed a rash for approximately 3 months and the area has now started to "drain." On physical exam, you note an erythematous, oozing, right nipple and areolar complex. There are no palpable breast masses and mammogram is normal. Which of the following treatments is appropriate?

- **A.** Topical steroids and 2-week follow-up
- **B.** Biopsy area of rash
- **C.** Wet-to-dry dressings
- **D.** Lanolin cream and 1-month follow-up
- **E.** Dermatology consult

The next two questions (items 36 and 37) correspond to the following vignette.

A 42-year-old female returns to your clinic for her annual breast exam. Three years ago the patient underwent a right breast, wide local excision, axillary lymph node dissection for an infiltrating ductal carcinoma diagnosis. All 14 of the lymph nodes were negative, and the patient underwent radiation treatment and was prescribed tamoxifen for 5 years. The patient reports that her health has been excellent, but she is concerned about a new area of fullness in her right breast. On exam you palpate a 2 cm area in her right breast. A mammogram is obtained that is concerning for malignancy. A needle core biopsy demonstrates infiltrating ductal carcinoma. A metastatic work-up is done; and all tests are negative.

36. What is the most appropriate treatment option?

A. Lumpectomy with whole-breast radiation
B. Modified radical mastectomy
C. Radiation therapy in combination with chemotherapy
D. Total mastectomy with postoperative radiation for positive chest wall margins and/or chemotherapy
E. Chemotherapy alone

37. Which of the following syndromes is associated with an increased risk of breast cancer?

A. Lynch syndrome
B. Li-Fraumeni syndrome
C. Brown-Séquard syndrome
D. Von Hippel-Lindau syndrome
E. Crow-Fukase syndrome
F. Beckwith-Wiedemann syndrome

End of set

The next two questions (items 38 and 39) correspond to the following vignette.

A 35-year-old female is referred to your clinic for a new breast lump. The patient tells you that she has done breast self-exams on a monthly basis for at least the last 3 years, and this past month she noticed a lump in her left breast. The patient also tells you that the mass changes in size and tenderness relative to her menstrual cycle. There has been no nipple discharge, and the patient has not had any recent unexpected weight loss. On physical exam, you note bilateral nodular breasts, and a dominant mass in the upper, outer quadrant of the left breast. There are no palpable axillary, supra, or infraclavicular nodes or breast skin changes. Mammography demonstrates dense breast tissue throughout without findings suggestive of malignancy.

38. The current screening guidelines for breast cancer recommend that all women should begin receiving annual mammograms at what age?

A. 35
B. 55
C. 40
D. 45
E. 50

39. The patient is very worried and prefers that you perform an excisional biopsy of the mass. This procedure is completed the following week. The pathology report states that the excised breast tissue is consistent with fibrocystic disease without any evidence of atypia, with lobular carcinoma in situ on the superior, medial margin of the specimen. What further treatment is indicated?

A. Re-excision of the positive margin
B. Modified radical mastectomy
C. Radiation therapy
D. Close observation
E. Axillary lymph node staging

End of set

The next two questions (items 40 and 41) correspond to the following vignette.

A 63-year-old male is seen in your clinic for evaluation of a CT-confirmed mass in the head of the pancreas that was found during a work-up for painless jaundice. You refer the patient for an ERCP, at which time brush biopsies are performed. These biopsies reveal adenocarcinoma. Based on the CT findings, the patient appears to have a resectable tumor and you recommend that he undergo a Whipple procedure.

40. What is the most common complication associated with the standard Whipple procedure that you should discuss with the patient?

A. Delayed gastric emptying
B. Pancreatic fistula
C. Wound infection
D. Bile leak
E. Pancreatitis

41. What is the most common location of a pancreatic adenocarcinoma?

A. Tail
B. Superior
C. Head
D. Body
E. Anterior

End of set

The next three questions (items 42–44) correspond to the following vignette.

A 44-year-old male presents to clinic after finding a small lump on the right side of his neck. The patient first noticed the lump 3 weeks ago and thought it would go away, but it has remained unchanged. The patient states that the lump is not painful, has no other symptoms, is otherwise healthy, takes no medications, and has had no prior surgeries. On physical exam, you note a well-developed male with a 2 cm nodule on the left lobe of the thyroid gland. No lymphadenopathy is appreciated elsewhere on exam, and the remainder of the physical exam is normal.

42. Which of the following is the most appropriate next step in obtaining a diagnosis?

A. CT scan of the neck
B. Fine-needle aspiration
C. Incisional biopsy
D. Lobectomy
E. Total thyroidectomy

43. After the correct procedure is performed, the pathology report reads as follows: "suspicious of papillary thyroid cancer." The patient is scheduled for surgery. In the operating room the mass is found to measure approximately 2 cm. What is the most appropriate surgical procedure for this patient?

A. Enucleation of the mass
B. Thyroid lobectomy
C. Thyroid lobectomy with isthmectomy
D. Subtotal thyroidectomy
E. Total thyroidectomy

44. Following surgery, the patient undergoes radio-iodine ablation and is subsequently started on thyroid hormone replacement therapy. Three years later, at a routine clinic visit with his primary care physician, a 1.5 cm firm cervical mass is noted. What laboratory test is most indicative of recurrent tumor?

A. Thyroid-stimulating hormone
B. Free T_4 level
C. Calcitonin
D. Thyroglobulin
E. T_3 reuptake level

End of set

The next two questions (items 45 and 46) correspond to the following vignette.

A 45-year-old male presents to your clinic complaining of abdominal pain. The patient states this pain has been present for the last 6 months, but it now occurs more frequently. He describes the pain as being dull, mainly localized to the epigastrium, radiating on occasion to the right upper quadrant. The pain also occurs during times of stress and fasting and is usually relieved after eating meals. The patient's father and brother both experience many of the same symptoms and have been treated for *Helicobacter pylori* infection in the past. The patient asks you whether such an infection might also be the source of his problem.

45. Which of the following is most often associated with *H. pylori* infection?

A. Gastric ulcer
B. Gastric lymphoma
C. Esophageal ulcer
D. Gastric carcinoma
E. Chronic NSAID use
F. Gastric maltoma

46. What is the usual initial therapy for patients with symptomatic *H. pylori* infection?

A. Bismuth subsalicylate and metronidazole
B. Parietal cell vagotomy
C. Proton pump inhibitors
D. H_2 blockers
E. Mucosal barrier drugs

End of set

---

47. A 54-year-old African American male presents to your clinic with a 3-month history of increasing difficulty with swallowing. The patient states that the difficulty initially began with only solid foods, but now he is also having trouble with liquids. Past medical history is remarkable for a myocardial infarction 4 years ago, a history of alcohol abuse, and a 1.5-pack-per-day smoking habit. Medications include metoprolol and aspirin. On review of systems the patient complains of a 14-pound weight loss over the last 2 months. Vitals signs and physical exam are unremarkable. What is the most appropriate next step in the evaluation of this patient?

A. Upper GI
B. Esophagram
C. Thoracic CT scan
D. Endoscopy
E. Enteroclysis

The next three questions (items 48–50) correspond to the following vignette.

A 45-year-old woman comes to your clinic to discuss cadaveric renal transplantation. The patient has polycystic kidney disease complicated by end-stage renal disease and is currently undergoing hemodialysis three times a week. The transplant team has evaluated the patient, and she has been placed on the transplant waiting list. You are seeing her for preoperative evaluation. During your discussion of the postoperative course, you explain that despite improved immunosuppressive drugs, rejection may still occur.

48. Which of the following descriptions characterizes acute rejection?

- **A.** Associated with a response to minor histocompatibility antigens
- **B.** Occurs rapidly, usually while in the operating room, and is treated by graft removal
- **C.** Is irreversible despite immunosuppressive therapy
- **D.** Primarily caused by a preexisting humoral response of preformed antibodies
- **E.** Mediated by cellular immunity with graft infiltration of small lymphocytes and mononuclear cells

49. Nine months after your initial clinic visit, the patient undergoes a cadaveric renal transplant and has an uncomplicated postoperative course. The patient is discharged from the hospital on an immunosuppressive regimen of mycophenolate mofetil (CellCept), tacrolimus (Prograf), and a steroid taper with a creatinine level of 1.2. Four weeks after her surgery, during a routine clinic visit, the patient tells you that she is urinating less, has had some weight gain, and is experiencing right lower extremity edema. Vital signs are as follows: T 37.1°C, HR 75, and BP 135/76. The patient, with clear breath sounds bilaterally, and the incision is healing nicely without erythema or drainage. On abdominal exam, the graft feels "boggy" and is slightly tender to palpation. Laboratory values are as follows: WBC 9000, HCT 35%, PLT 100,000, Na 140 mmol/L, K 4.3 mmol/L, Cl 109 mmol/L, HCO_3 22 mmol/L, BUN 46 mg/dL, creatinine 2.5 mg/dL, and a Prograf level in therapeutic range. A US is obtained (Figure 49). What is the most appropriate next step in the management of this patient?

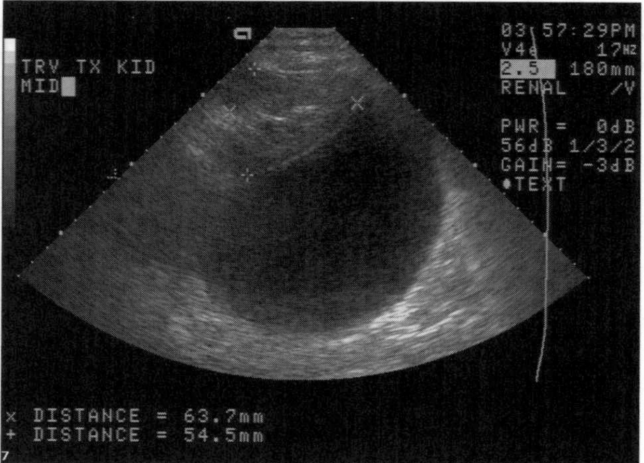

Figure 49 • Image courtesy of the University of Utah School of Medicine, Salt Lake City, Utah.

A. Aspiration of fluid collection for culture and chemistry analysis
B. Reduction of immunosuppressive regimen
C. Percutaneous transplant graft biopsy
D. Prompt increase in immunosuppression to treat acute rejection
E. Reevaluation in 1 week to assess for absorption of fluid collection

50. At the 6-month postoperative clinic visit, the patient complains of pain and pruritus of her back. Vital signs are as follows: T 37.5°C, HR 67, and BP 135/85. On physical exam, you notice an erythematous, papulovesicular rash in a well-defined strip across the right side of the patient's back. Some of the lesions contain scabs. The remainder of the exam is normal. Laboratory values are as follows: WBC 5000, HCT 39%, PLT 120,000, Na 139 mmol/L, K 3.5 mmol/L, Cl 102 mmol/L, HCO_3 24 mmol/L, BUN 12 mg/dL, creatinine 1.0 mg/dL, glucose 99 mg/dL, and Prograf level in therapeutic range. A chest x-ray is normal. What is the most appropriate treatment?

A. Oral acyclovir and follow-up in clinic
B. A reduction in immunosuppressive medications
C. Hospital admission, IV followed by oral acyclovir, and a reduction in the immunosuppressive regimen
D. An increase in the immunosuppressive regimen
E. Close observation

End of set

Block

ONE Answers and Explanations

Block

ONE

Answer Key

1. D
2. B
3. D
4. C
5. B
6. D
7. B
8. C
9. A
10. C
11. C
12. C
13. C
14. B
15. D
16. E
17. E
18. C
19. D
20. E
21. D
22. B
23. B
24. C
25. A
26. D
27. B
28. A
29. E
30. D
31. A
32. E
33. A
34. E
35. B
36. D
37. B
38. C
39. D
40. A
41. C
42. B
43. E
44. D
45. A
46. A
47. D
48. E
49. A
50. C

1. **D.** Crohn's disease is a chronic inflammatory disorder of the alimentary tract and can be rapidly progressive or indolent in its course, with a currently unknown etiology. This disease tends to involve transmural inflammation not limited to the mucosa and submucosa like ulcerative colitis. It occurs most commonly between the ages of 15 and 35 years. Most patients present with abdominal pain, weight loss, and diarrhea. Symptoms have usually been present for 2 to 3 years before the diagnosis is confirmed. Intermittent exacerbations are marked by aphthous ulcers, granulomas, and transmural chronic inflammation with fissures and fistulas. Differences between Crohn's disease and ulcerative colitis are demonstrated in Table 1.

A, B, C, E. Sclerosing cholangitis, rectal involvement, treatment via ileoanal pouch procedure, and rectal bleeding are all consistent with ulcerative colitis.

TABLE 1 Crohn's Disease versus Ulcerative Colitis

Crohn's Disease	Ulcerative Colitis
Gross Appearance	
Transmural involvement	Mucosal involvement
Segmental disease	Continuous disease beginning in the rectum
Thickened bowel wall	Normal thickness of bowel wall
Creeping fat	
Pseudopolyps rare	Pseudopolyps common
Any section of the alimentary tract may be involved	Limited to the colon with rare small-bowel involvement
Perianal disease common	Perianal disease uncommon
Histological Appearance	
Crypt abscesses uncommon	Crypt abscesses common
Granulomas present	Granulomas absent
Cobblestoning	No cobblestoning
Fistulas	No fistulas
Pseudopolyps absent	Pseudopolyps present
Deep, narrow longitudinal ulcers	Shallow wide ulcers

2. **B.** Medical treatment focuses on immunosuppression with a variety of immunosuppressive medications, such as corticosteroids, sulfasalazine, metronidazole, azathioprine, 6-mercaptopurine, methotrexate, and cyclosporine. Surgical therapy is reserved for complications, including obstruction, bleeding, fistulas, perforation, abscesses, and cancer. The most common cause of obstruction is intraluminal strictures. Small-bowel strictures, like that seen in the abdominal CT (note arrow in Figure 2B), are a complication of transmural involvement. Resections of these segments would eventually lead to short bowel syndrome. Stricturoplasty is effective at relieving obstructive symptoms without adverse sequelae.

A. Adhesions would be an extremely rare cause of obstruction because the patient has not had any prior abdominal surgery.

C. Volvulus is more likely a cause of large-bowel obstruction. It is usually seen in older, debilitated patients. The CT scan obtained demonstrates a small-bowel stricture, not a volvulus.

D. Femoral hernias are more prone to becoming incarcerated, thereby causing obstructive symptoms. The femoral-inguinal area should be thoroughly investigated in anyone with symptoms of bowel obstruction. This patient's clinical picture and CT are most consistent with a Crohn's stricture, however.

E. Intra-abdominal infection may lead to ileus. The CT shows a Crohn's induced stricture, not a pelvic abscess.

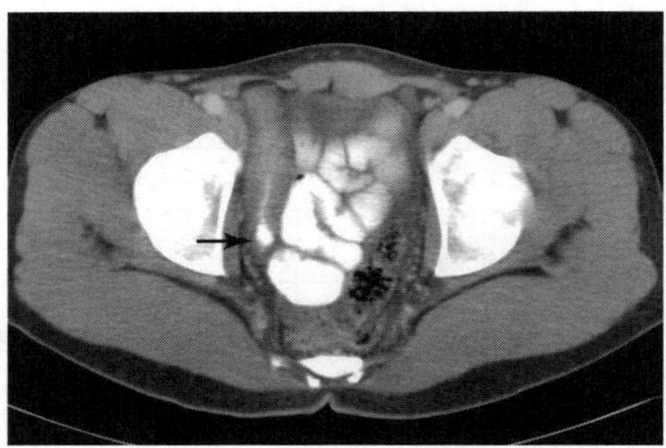

Figure 2B • Image courtesy of the University of Utah School of Medicine, Salt Lake City, Utah.

3. **D.** Extra-intestinal manifestations of inflammatory bowel disease (IBD) include aphthous ulcers, pyoderma gangrenosum, iritis, erythema nodosum, sclerosing cholangitis, arthritis, ankylosing spondylitis, and kidney disease. Answers A, B, C, and E are all intestinal manifestations of inflammatory bowel disease.

A. Abdominal pain is more common in Crohn's disease than in ulcerative colitis (UC) but can be seen in both conditions.

B. The risk of carcinoma of the involved bowel is an intestinal manifestation linked to both UC and Crohn's disease.

C, E. Bowel wall thickening is an intestinal manifestation of Crohn's disease, along with creeping fat, segmental involvement, linear ulcers, and lymphoid aggregation.

4. **C.** This patient has primary sclerosing cholangitis (PSC), which is an idiopathic disorder of the biliary tree. Approximately 50% to 70% of cases are associated with inflammatory bowel disease, most commonly with ulcerative colitis. The risk of PSC remains, even after having a total colectomy. This disease causes multiple intrahepatic and extrahepatic strictures of the bile ducts and is best diagnosed by ERCP. It usually has a characteristic "string of beads" appearance as seen in Figure 4 (note arrows).

A. There is no indication for an exploratory laparotomy prior to an appropriate work-up.

B, D. Obtaining either a CT or an MRI of the abdomen is not the preferred way to visualize the biliary tree in this setting.

E. A colonoscopy will not add to the work-up of PSC.

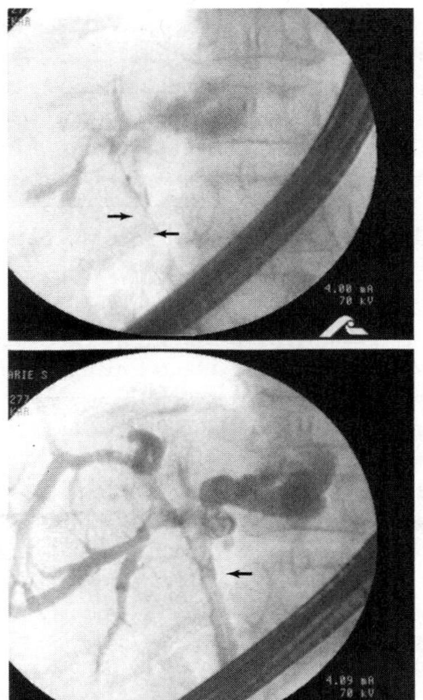

Figure 4 • Image courtesy of the University of Utah School of Medicine, Salt Lake City, Utah.

5. B. PSC is chronic and necessitates a liver transplant in the majority of cases.

A, D. This disease usually involves the entire biliary tree, and removal of only the gallbladder will not address the underlying problem.

C. Although choledochojejunostomy may temporize the complications from extrahepatic involvement, this disease is chronic and progressive. The biliary tree would not be effectively decompressed over the long term by such a procedure.

E. The Whipple procedure is indicated for pathology involving the head of the pancreas, ampulla of Vater, and duodenum. It would not affect the biliary sclerosis seen in this case.

6. **D.** Hypercalcemia is caused by a variety of disease processes. The most common etiology in an outpatient setting is primary hyperparathyroidism, whereas in hospitalized patients the most common cause is cancer. Other causes include thiazide diuretics, Paget's disease, vitamins D and A toxicity, sarcoidosis, and milk alkali syndrome. The signs and symptoms of primary hyperparathyroidism are most commonly remembered by the mnemonic "stones, bones, groans, and psychiatric overtones." ECG findings consist of prolonged PR interval with a shortened QT interval. These patients usually present with dehydration, which can be severe in a calcemic crisis as is seen with this patient. The most appropriate initial treatment consists of IV fluid hydration with normal saline.

A, C. A serum PTH level and Sestamibi scan should be used once the patient is stabilized to help identify the source of hypercalcemia.

B, E. Once initial treatment is accomplished, furosemide may be used to reduce the serum calcium level through diuresis. Plicamycin (Mithramycin) may be also used in follow-up treatment for causes of hypercalcemia due to a malignancy.

7. **B.** In primary hyperparathyroidism, both calcium and PTH levels are increased, usually due to continued PTH secretion from a parathyroid adenoma. Oversecretion of PTH causes abnormal fluxes of calcium in bone, the kidneys, and the GI tract, resulting in hypercalcemia, hypercalciuria, and increased bone turnover. Serum phosphate level is lowered due to PTH effects on phosphate excretion from the kidney. Although most patients with primary hyperparathyroidism are asymptomatic, as many as 50% will experience subtle neurobehavioral symptoms such as fatigue and weakness ("psychiatric overtones"), 20% will have a history of nephrolithiasis ("stones"), and rarely patients will present with bone pain ("bones" and "groans").

A. A high PTH level with low or low normal calcium and high serum phosphate levels is most consistent with secondary hyperparathyroidism seen in chronic renal failure. Secondary hyperparathyroidism is caused by low calcium levels, which, in turn, are caused by hypophosphatemia and decreased production of 1,25-dihydroxyvitamin D_2. Severe secondary hyperparathyroidism is an indication for parathyroidectomy if treatment with oral calcium and vitamin D is inadequate.

C. A decreased PTH level is not consistent with primary hyperparathyroidism.

D. Decreased PTH and calcium levels are not consistent with primary hyperparathyroidism, but may be seen with hypoparathyroidism due to damage to all parathyroid glands at surgery, parathyroid agenesis (DiGeorge syndrome), or autoimmune hypoparathyroidism as part of an autoimmune polyendocrinopathy candidiasis ectodermal dystrophy syndrome.

E. Normal levels of serum calcium, phosphate, and PTH are not consistent with the most likely diagnosis of primary hyperparathyroidism.

8. **C.** Patients should undergo cystoscopy with directed deep biopsies of suspicious lesions and multiple random biopsies of both the bladder and the prostatic urethra to confirm and stage the disease.

A. Urine culture is a nonspecific test obtained routinely to evaluate hematuria.

B. Patients suspected of having bladder cancer should eventually undergo an intravenous pyelogram (IVP) to rule out coincident upper urinary tract disease, but an IVP is not specific enough to evaluate a patient for bladder cancer.

D. Bladder washings for cytology would help confirm the diagnosis of bladder cancer, but will not locate or stage the disease.

E. Patients should undergo CT scan of the abdomen and pelvis—not MRI—to rule out metastatic disease and nodal involvement.

9. **A.** Transitional tumors account for approximately 90% of all bladder tumors. Approximately 70% of transitional tumors are superficial; the other 30% are invasive or metastatic. Patients in whom the tumor does not invade past the lamina propria do not typically receive adjuvant therapy. Patients with TA and T1 tumors (not invading past the lamina propria) who may be candidates for adjuvant intravesicular chemotherapy include those with high-grade lesions, aneuploid tumors, tumors greater than 5 cm in size, and those with persistently positive cytology. Such patients require close follow-up, because as many as 50% will develop recurrent disease. When recurrence does develop, it is usually at the same stage as the primary tumor.

B, C, D, E. See the explanation for A.

10. **C.** The next step in the work-up of this lung mass is to obtain a tissue biopsy. Definitive diagnosis and staging of the mass are the keys to this patient's management. Because this case involves a centrally located tumor, bronchoscopy with transbronchial biopsy is the most appropriate next step.

A. Waiting 6 months while looking for advancement of the tumor is not a viable option, because early diagnosis and therapy are key factors in improving survival, particularly with a centrally located mass that may progress to unresectable disease.

B. Because this case involves a centrally located tumor, it would be extremely difficult to biopsy the mass under CT guidance.

D. Mediastinoscopy is indicated for diagnosis if there is CT evidence of lymphadenopathy. With no evidence of a mediastinal mass, mediastinoscopy would be used for staging after diagnosis of a primary lung tumor.

E. Thoracoscopy with biopsy is more easily used in peripherally located masses in the lung.

11. **C.** Four types of primary lung tumors exist: adenocarcinoma, squamous cell carcinoma, small cell carcinoma, and large cell carcinoma. Small cell carcinoma (oat cell carcinoma) usually originates in the major bronchus near the hilum. It is known for its rapid growth and early metastasis to both lymphatic and blood vessels. It is therefore considered by many to be metastatic at the time of diagnosis.

A. Squamous cell carcinoma accounts for 30% of primary malignant lung tumors. It occurs centrally in the segmental, lobar, or mainstem bronchi. Slow growing and late to metastasize, this type of tumor lends itself to resection if diagnosed early enough.

B. Adenocarcinoma accounts for 40% of malignant lung tumors. It is most often peripheral in location. Like squamous cell carcinoma, adenocarcinoma is late to metastasize and may be resectable.

D. Ten percent of malignant lung tumors involve large cell carcinomas, which are also usually located in the periphery. These tumors show rapid growth and early metastasis, but are known to be less aggressive than small cell carcinomas. The majority of large cell carcinomas are poorly differentiated adenocarcinomas.

E. Hodgkin's disease is a lymphoma that usually presents with asymptomatic adenopathy and constitutional symptoms of fever, night sweats, and weight loss. Hodgkin's lymphomas are highly responsive to radiation and chemotherapy.

12. **C.** The most likely ectopically produced hormone by squamous cell carcinoma is parathyroid hormone or PTH-like peptide production, leading to hypercalcemia.

A. SIADH is mainly associated with small cell lung cancer.

B. Eaton-Lambert is a neurologic-myopathic syndrome that presents with symptoms similar to myasthenia gravis. This paraneoplastic syndrome is most commonly associated with small cell lung cancer.

D. Cushing's syndrome (ectopic ACTH production) is mainly associated with small cell lung cancer.

E. Ectopic acromegaly is associated with carcinoid tumors of the bronchus, pancreatic islet tumors, and cancers of the lung, breast, colon, and adrenal glands.

13. **C.** The Child-Pugh classification of cirrhosis is a method of predicting operative mortality. Patients with cirrhosis are at increased risk for associated morbidity and mortality for any kind of surgery. The operative mortality associated with Child's classes A, B, and C are 2%, 10%, and 50%, respectively. Score A is 5–6, score B is 7–9, and score C is 10 points or higher. See Table 13 for the relevant calculation.

A, B, D, E. Age, history of smoking, ALT and AST levels, and PTT are not used to determine the Child's classification.

TABLE 13 Child-Pugh Classification Points

Factor/Points	1	2	3
Serum bilirubin (mg/dL)	<2	2–3	>3
Serum albumin (g/dL)	>3.5	2.8–3.5	<2.8
Ascites	Absent	Mild	Moderate
Hepatic encephalopathy grade	None	1, 2	3, 4
PT (INR)	<1.7	1.7–2.3	>2.3

14. **B.** A patient with Child's class B cirrhosis and multiple co-morbidities is a poor operative candidate at risk for a significant mortality rate. A transjugular intrahepatic portosystemic shunt (TIPSS) is a radiologically guided, percutaneously placed shunt that decompresses the portal venous system to the systemic venous system. It is used in patients who are poor operative candidates, as well as sometimes for sustaining patients who are awaiting a transplant.

A, C, D. The mesocaval shunt, splenorenal shunt, and end-to-side shunt are all portal venous decompressive shunts that require an operative procedure and carry a high mortality rate in a patient with advanced cirrhosis.

E. A patient with Child's class B cirrhosis may eventually be an appropriate candidate for a liver transplant, but in this clinical situation it would not be the best option.

15. **D.** This is the classic description of hypertrophic pyloric stenosis. Patients present with a history of projectile emesis and often have a palpable, olive-shaped mass in the right upper quadrant. The contrast study images (note the arrows in Figures 15C and 15D) show the classic gastric outlet obstruction of pyloric stenosis. It is four times more common in male infants and usually presents at 4 to 8 weeks of age. Nonbilious vomiting that increases in volume and frequency is often seen. Dehydration is often seen with a hypokalemic, hypochloremic metabolic alkalosis. All resulting electrolyte abnormalities should be corrected prior to proceeding to the operating room. The Fredet-Ramstedt pyloromyotomy is the classic operation performed. Most patients resume oral intake within 12 hours of surgery.

A. Duodenal atresia presents as bilious emesis in the newborn and is associated with the classic "double bubble" sign on abdominal x-rays.

B. Cholangiocarcinoma is a tumor of the biliary tree; it is not typically seen in children.

C. Hirschsprung's disease presents as a relative colonic obstruction and difficulty passing stool due to an aganglionic segment of the distal colon.

E. Intestinal malrotation is a surgical emergency and must be considered. Infants with malrotation might vomit, however, they would also have distention and pain, which are symptoms not usually found in children with pyloric stenosis.

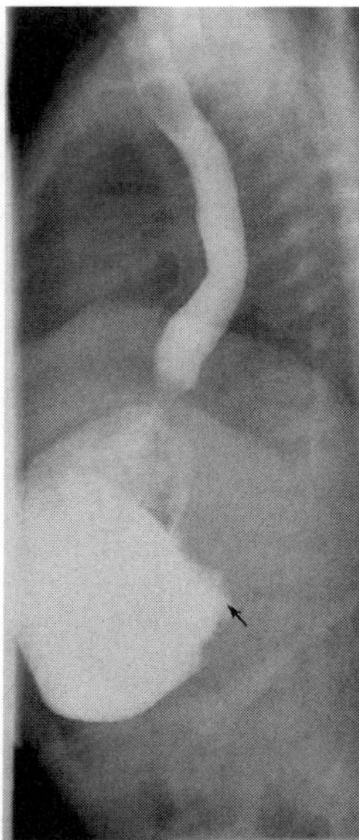

Figure 15C • Image courtesy of the University of Utah School of Medicine, Salt Lake City, Utah.

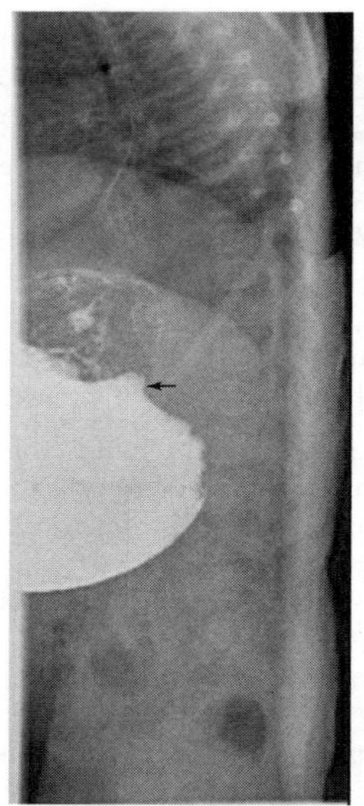

Figure 15D • Image courtesy of the University of Utah School of Medicine, Salt Lake City, Utah.

16. **E.** All incarcerated or strangulated hernias are considered a surgical emergency and should be repaired immediately. Reducible hernias may be repaired on an elective basis. All symptomatic hernias should be repaired with the exception of umbilical hernias in children younger than 4 years of age and adults with severe medical problems such as cirrhosis with ascites.

A. Incarceration of a hernia can lead to ischemia (strangulation) of the contents. Immediate treatment—not reevaluation—is needed. This patient needs to go to the operating room to reduce and repair his hernia and determine whether resection of ischemic bowel is needed.

B, C, D. Nothing found on ultrasound, CT, or upper GI imaging with SBFT would influence the plan for immediate exploration.

17. **E.** This patient has a urinary tract infection (UTI) secondary to benign prostatic hypertrophy (BPH). The main symptoms of BPH are categorized as obstructive and irritative voiding symptoms. They are caused by hyperplastic growth of prostatic adenoma in the transition zone of the prostate. BPH is the most common cause of bladder outlet obstruction in men more than 50 years old. Complications include urinary retention, UTIs, bladder stones secondary to stasis, and even renal failure secondary to high-pressure urinary retention. Medical management of BPH includes the use of alpha antagonists (terazosin) to decrease smooth muscle tone and 5-alpha-reductase blockade (finasteride) to inhibit the conversion of testosterone to dihydrotestosterone. If medical therapy is unsuccessful, the surgical treatment is transurethral resection of the prostate (TURP). This patient should also be treated with a course of antibiotics for his UTI.

A. Gonorrhea, a sexually transmitted disease, may cause many of these symptoms and should be included on the differential diagnosis. However, purulent urethral discharge is usually present with this STD.

B. Although a UTI may be present, prostate cancer usually occurs in the peripheral zones of the prostate and does not cause bladder outlet obstruction.

C. Bladder stones, compared to kidney stones, are more likely to cause a UTI. Kidney stones usually result in severe flank pain that radiates into the groin.

D. Although hydronephrosis may be present, it is also a result of bladder obstruction due to BPH.

F. Rectal cancer often presents with rectal bleeding upon bowel movements (hematochezia), alteration in bowel habits, feeling of painful incomplete evacuation (tenesmus), and an intrarectal palpable tumor on rectal exam. Presentation with primarily urinary symptoms would not be the case with rectal cancer.

18. **C.** Risk factors that are significant for developing prostate cancer include older age, African ancestry, a positive family history, high dietary fat intake, and cadmium found in cigarette smoke. Unlike most cancers, prostate cancer does not have a peak age of incidence, but its incidence continues to increase with increasing age. Family history is a risk factor, with the age at which the relative was diagnosed being the most significant issue. For example, if the relative was diagnosed at age 70, the patient's relative risk is increased fourfold; this risk increases sevenfold if the relative was diagnosed at age 50. A high fat intake may increase the risk of prostate cancer by almost a factor of two. Cadmium, found in cigarette smoke, alkaline batteries, and the welding industry, adds to the risk of prostate cancer. Prostate cancer is the most common malignancy affecting men and is the second leading cause of cancer-related death.

A, D. Prostate cancer is the second leading cause of cancer-related death.

B. African ancestry is a risk factor, with African American patients typically presenting at a later stage of disease as compared to Caucasians.

E. The majority of patients with prostate cancer are asymptomatic. Symptoms suggest the presence of locally advanced or metastatic disease.

19. **D.** Cryptorchidism is the failure of normal testicular descent during embryologic development. Its incidence is 1% to 2% in full-term infants and as much as 30% in preterm infants. Placement of the testis into the scrotal sac is indicated after age 1 but prior to age 2. If the testis has not descended into the scrotum by age 1, surgery is indicated to place the testicle in the scrotum. Undescended testes will continue to secrete androgens, but spermatogenic function is progressively impaired. Scrotal placement of the testes should occur prior to age 2 to preserve spermatogenic function. If the testes are not able to be placed successfully into the scrotum, orchiectomy is indicated due to the significantly increased risk of testicular cancer (30 times greater) if the testes are left in an intra-abdominal position.

A, B. An ultrasound or CT scan would not change the course of management, as described in the explanation for D.

C. After age 2, orchiectomy is indicated due to the increased risk of cancer and spermatogenic failure.

E. Waiting until age 4 would add to the risks of both spermatogenic failure and risk of testicular cancer.

20. **E.** A perirectal abscess must be widely opened and drained to heal. Intravenous antibiotics are likewise indicated, but the definitive treatment of the abscess remains surgical drainage. If left undrained, the abscess may progress to a perineal soft tissue infection, especially in immunocompromised patients or in individuals with poorly controlled diabetes. If the abscess recurs after being drained, one should suspect an underlying fistula or ischiorectal abscess.

A. While admission and IV antibiotics are appropriate therapy, the definitive treatment is surgical drainage.

B. Needle drainage is not adequate management and does not allow for debridement of necrotic tissue.

C. Because the fluctuant mass is easily palpable and the extent will be defined during your exploration of the wound, localization via CT is not needed prior to primary drainage.

D. As in the explanation for C, evaluation using endorectal ultrasound is not needed prior to initial drainage.

21. **D.** Approximately 50% of perirectal abscesses will develop a fistula communicating with the anal crypt.

A, B, C, E. Even in a high-risk diabetic patient, anal incontinence, colovesical fistula, anal stricture, and anal fissure are all much less likely to occur.

22. **B.** Ductal carcinoma in situ, also known as intraductal carcinoma, is a premalignant lesion. It is most often found on mammography as microcalcifications. Because it may subsequently develop into infiltrating ductal carcinoma of the breast, surgical treatment is required. Note the arrow and blocked marking of the microcalcifications on Figure 22.

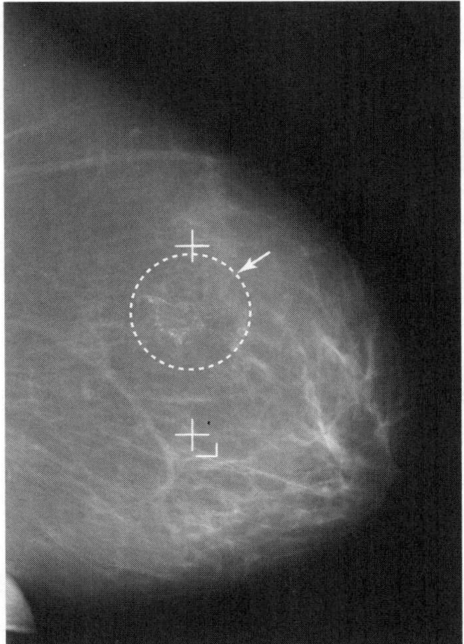

Figure 22 • Image courtesy of the University of Utah School of Medicine, Salt Lake City, Utah.

A. DCIS is usually nonpalpable and is primarily found on mammography, rather than on physical exam.

C. The risk of metastasis to lymph nodes is less than 2%, so an axillary dissection is usually not done with the surgical treatment of DCIS.

D. Local treatment of the whole breast is required for DCIS. This is accomplished by lumpectomy and whole-breast radiation, or with a modified radical mastectomy.

E. The chance of lymph node involvement is only 2%, as this condition is usually seen as microinvasion.

23. **B.** This clinical scenario and CT scan (see the arrow in Figure 23B) are characteristic of amebic abscess of the liver, caused by *Entamoeba histolytica*, which typically occurs in young men who have emigrated from or recently traveled to an endemic area. Symptoms most often include pain in the right upper quadrant, fever, and anorexia. Diagnosis is confirmed with an indirect hemagglutination test with titers greater than 1:512. The CT scan demonstrates the abscess as a single hypodense lesion within the liver.

A. An elevated alkaline phosphate level (liver function test) is most often present with amebic abscess, but it is nonspecific to this disease.

C. Leukocytosis and anemia are often present with amebic abscess and are nonspecific findings found in a complete blood count test.

D. An indirect Coomb's test is usually obtained to rule out a hemolytic reaction caused by antibodies in the patient's serum.

E. A chemistry panel is a very nonspecific test for an amebic abscess.

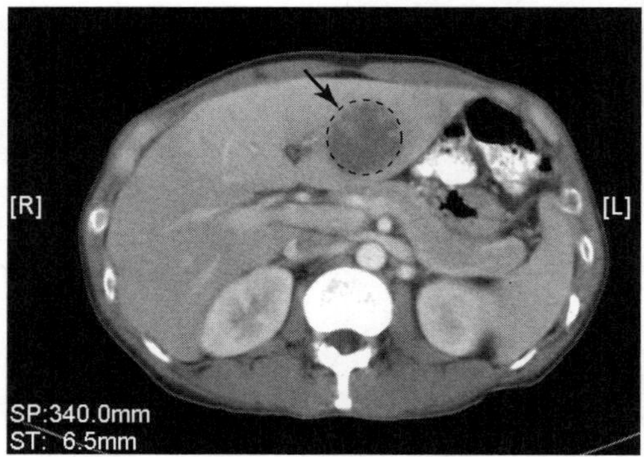

Figure 23B • Image courtesy of the University of Utah School of Medicine, Salt Lake City, Utah.

24. **C.** Initial treatment of an amebic abscess is oral metronidazole, which cures approximately 75% of patients. Drainage of the abscess is reserved for patients who fail initial therapy.

A. Percutaneous drainage is reserved for those who fail an initial trial of oral metronidazole.

B. Operative drainage would be reserved for patients who do not respond to oral metronidazole and percutaneous drainage.

D, E. The antibiotic regimen of gentamicin, ampicillin, and metronidazole is more appropriate for a pyogenic abscess of the liver.

25. **A.** Hemangiomas are the most common benign masses found in the liver. They are of vascular origin and may be associated with pain in the right upper quadrant, bruits, shock with bleeding, or high-output heart failure. Hepatic hemangiomas are usually found incidentally on CT scan. Biopsy should not generally be performed due to the risk of hemorrhage. Figure 25B is a CT scan showing a hepatic hemangioma (note arrow). Notice its hypervascularity compared to the surrounding hepatic parenchyma.

B. Although a hamartoma is a possibility, hemangiomas are the most common benign tumors of the liver.

C. The patient's labs are within normal limits with a negative work-up for hepatic cancer.

D. A bacterial abscess is unlikely because the patient is afebrile, without any prior intra-abdominal infections.

E. A hydatid cyst is unlikely because the patient has not traveled to endemic areas.

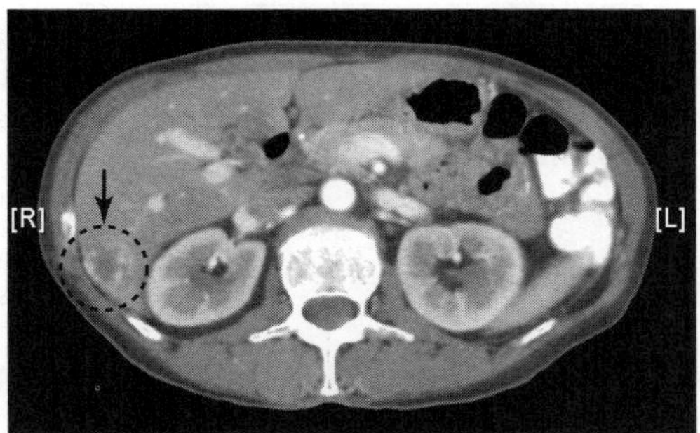

Figure 25B • Image courtesy of the University of Utah School of Medicine, Salt Lake City, Utah.

26. **D.** Observation is the treatment of choice for asymptomatic hepatic hemangiomas less than 5 cm in diameter.

A. A hepatic wedge resection would be a reasonable choice if the patient was having symptoms or if the lesion was greater than 5 cm.

B. Percutaneous drainage is contraindicated due to possible hemorrhage.

C. Hepatic lobectomy would be an option with multiple symptomatic hemangiomas.

E. Sclerotherapy is not currently a treatment option for this disease.

27. **B.** Although relatively rare, hepatocellular carcinoma (HCC) is one of the most lethal solid tumors in the world. Many different risk factors are associated with it, with the most common cause throughout the world being chronic hepatitis B infection.

A. Polyvinyl chloride (PVC), nitrites, and hydrocarbons have all been implicated as hepatic carcinogens.

C. The hepatitis A virus does not cause chronic hepatitis, so it is not associated with an increased risk of developing HCC.

D. Alcohol-related cirrhosis is the leading cause of HCC in the United States, Canada, and Western Europe.

E. Aflatoxins are secondary fungal metabolites that frequently contaminate foods. Exposure to them is associated with development of HCC.

28. **A.** Appendiceal carcinoid tumors at the tip of the appendix that are less than 2 cm in size require appendectomy only. For tumors at the base of the appendix or those greater than 2 cm, a right hemicolectomy is advocated. Unfortunately, carcinoid tumors have minimal clinical manifestations until metastases have occurred. Treatment for carcinoid tumors depends on the tumor location and size. Treatment of metastatic disease often consists of palliative care for the symptoms of carcinoid syndrome.

B. The role of radiation therapy in the treatment of carcinoid tumors involving metastatic disease, such as in this scenario, is limited to palliation of painful bone metastases. It is not indicated in cases of metastases to the liver.

C. Surgical resection of hepatic metastases would be considered if they are located in surgically accessible areas of the liver.

D. Observation alone is an incorrect course of action. The prognosis for malignant carcinoid syndrome is good compared to other malignancies.

E. Trastuzumab (Herceptin) is a monoclonal antibody used as a chemotherapeutic agent and approved for use in HER-2 neu-positive metastatic breast cancer.

29. **E.** Carcinoid syndrome classically presents with flushing (95% of cases), diarrhea (80%), valvular heart disease (40%), and wheezing (20%). Carcinoid tumors secrete serotonin, which is responsible for the symptoms of the syndrome. The systemic effects of the disease do not present until metastatic disease occurs in the liver (Figure 29), which filters serotonin. With metastases, some active serotonin passes directly into the central circulation, causing the previously mentioned syndrome. Common sites of tumors include the appendix (most common), ileum, rectum, and bronchi.

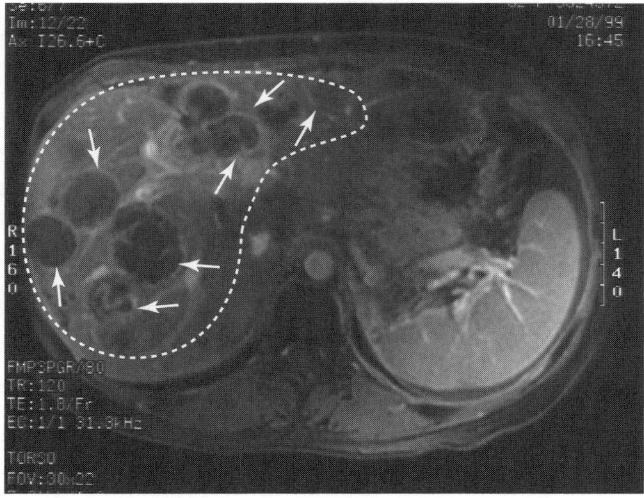

Figure 29 • Image courtesy of the University of Utah School of Medicine, Salt Lake City, Utah.

A. Adenocarcinoma is not associated with the signs and symptoms described here.

B. Insulinoma symptoms usually present as Whipple's triad: hypoglycemic symptoms produced by fasting, blood glucose less than 50 mg/dL during symptomatic attacks, and relief of symptoms by administration of glucose.

C. Lymphoma usually presents with constitutional symptoms such as fever, night sweats, and malaise.

D. Gastrinoma usually presents with symptoms of peptic ulcers, diarrhea, weight loss, and abdominal pain.

30. **D.** The classic lab test to diagnose carcinoid syndrome is serum serotonin or a 24-hour urinary 5-hydroxyindoleacetic acid (5-HIAA) level.

A. Serum gastrin is used to diagnose a gastrinoma.

B. Serum protein C is a helpful test in diagnosing an insulinoma.

C. A colonoscopy would help determine whether the lesion in the liver was due to colorectal cancer.

E. Obtaining urinary metanepherines is important in the diagnosis of pheochromocytomas.

31. **A.** This patient has a perianal abscess that appears to have spontaneously drained. Perianal abscesses most often arise from obstruction of an anal gland that becomes infected and overgrown with bacteria. These glands are located between the internal and external anal sphincters. If the infection tracks down this space toward the skin, a perianal abscess occurs. Because this abscess has drained spontaneously and has left an open cavity, it is safe to simply begin wound care with wet-to-dry dressing changes.

B. Rectal irrigations are inadequate therapy for an abscess. The drained abscess needs to be treated with aggressive wound care.

C. Antibiotics are used if significant cellulitis is present or the patient is immunocompromised, but not as the only treatment.

D. Incision and drainage of a perianal abscess are the proper management. In this case, however, the abscess has already drained spontaneously and no further drainage is required, unless there is evidence of grossly necrotic tissue.

E. Warm sitz baths alone will not adequately treat this type of infection. They can be employed postoperatively to assist with hygiene of the drained area.

32. **E.** The upper one-third of the anus originates from endoderm, with the lower two-thirds originating from ectoderm. The dentate line marks this transition point. It is important surgically as the embryologic origin determines the blood supply, innervation, and lymphatic drainage.

A. The innervation above the dentate line is autonomic; the innervation below it is somatic.

B. Stratified squamous epithelium lines the lumen below the dentate line, whereas columnar epithelium lines the lumen above it.

C. The blood supply above the dentate line originates from the superior rectal artery, a branch of the inferior mesenteric artery that originates from the aorta. The arterial supply below the dentate line originates from the inferior rectal artery, a branch of the internal pudendal artery that originates from the internal iliac artery. The venous system follows the arterial system.

D. A transanal biopsy and excision of benign and malignant tumors are possible well above the dentate line.

F. Lymphatic drainage above the dentate line flows into the lymph nodes along the iliac vessels. These eventually drain into the peri-aortic lymph nodes. Lymphatic drainage below the line goes to the inguinal lymph nodes.

33. **A.** This patient has a proximal bowel obstruction due to the bilious output. It is important to rule out any type of volvulus, which could potentially compromise blood flow to the bowel. The most appropriate study in this setting is upper GI imaging, which would define the location of the obstruction. Such a study will demonstrate distention of the duodenum, abnormal positioning of the duodenojejunal segment (to the right of the midline), and a narrowing (bird's beak) at the point of obstruction.

B. Upper endoscopy is not indicated in this scenario, as it would not be helpful in ruling out a midgut volvulus.

C. A barium enema is helpful to evaluate distal obstructions, but it is not helpful in case of a proximal obstruction. It may show abnormal positioning of the cecum in the right upper quadrant consistent with malrotation of the intestine.

D. Exploratory laparotomy is indicated in an emergency only in the setting of a midgut volvulus. Because the child has no peritoneal signs, further elucidation of his abdominal pain should be sought prior to emergent surgery.

E. Colonoscopy is not helpful, as it visualizes only the colon and not the proximal small bowel.

34. **E.** An intestinal malrotation may result in intestinal obstruction with vascular compromise and is a surgical emergency. Treatment involves exploring the abdomen, untwisting the bowel, and performing lyses of adhesions, also known as Ladd's procedure.

A. Endoscopy has no role in the management of intestinal malrotation complicated by volvulus.

B. Although patients with intestinal malrotation require fluid resuscitation, observation is inappropriate because delay in surgical intervention can result in infarction of the bowel.

C. A Gastrografin enema may help relieve the obstruction caused by meconium plug syndrome. Unfortunately, it is not helpful in this clinical scenario.

D. Air-contrast enemas are diagnostic and therapeutic in children with intussusception.

35. **B.** All suspicious skin lesions warrant a biopsy. In this case, the patient presents with classic symptoms of Paget's disease of the breast. This disease presents as an eczematous lesion of the nipple-areolar complex associated with itching or burning, as well as possibly erosion and ulceration. A biopsy will demonstrate Paget cells, consisting of invasion of the epidermis by invasive ductal carcinoma. Paget's disease occurs in less than 1% of all breast cancers. Surgical treatment involves a modified radical mastectomy or breast conservation with excision of the nipple areolar complex and breast radiation.

A. Treatment with topical steroids will merely delay the time until an appropriate biopsy can be obtained.

C. Like steroid use, use of dressings or antibiotic creams will merely delay the diagnosis.

D. Lanolin or other creams that will soothe the area will merely delay the diagnosis.

E. Unfortunately, Paget's carcinoma of the breast is frequently misdiagnosed and initially treated as dermatitis or infection, leading to a delay in its diagnosis. Any suspicious skin lesion of the breast should be biopsied.

36. **D.** Women who have undergone previous breast conservation therapy for breast cancer have a 5% to 10% risk of local recurrence at 10 years. These patients should undergo complete restaging of this new diagnosis. Those patients with purely local recurrence should undergo a mastectomy followed by radiation therapy for positive chest wall margins. Chemotherapy is given based on tumor characteristics.

A. This patient has failed initial breast conservation treatment and must now undergo a mastectomy, not repeat lumpectomy.

B. This patient has previously undergone an axillary node dissection. Most cases will not need a repeat axillary dissection.

C. Given the scenario presented, this patient requires further surgical excision for local control.

E. Isolated local recurrence may be treated without systemic chemotherapy. Mastectomy is the most effective measure for local control.

37. **B.** Li-Fraumeni syndrome is an autosomal dominant disorder caused by mutation of the p53 tumor suppressor gene; it is associated with increased incidence of breast cancer. A diagnosis of Li-Fraumeni syndrome is made when all of the following characteristics are present in a family: a sarcoma diagnosis in a person younger than 45 years of age; a first-degree relative with cancer at less than 45 years of age; and a first- or second-degree relative with cancer at age less than 45 years or sarcoma at any age. Approximately 70% of Li-Fraumeni cases are the result of mutations in p53, a gene on chromosome 17. Mutations in p53 confer an increased risk for early-onset breast cancer, childhood sarcoma, osteosarcoma, brain tumors, leukemia, and adrenocortical carcinoma. Individuals with a p53 mutation have a 50% chance of developing one of the associated cancers by age 50. Women with this syndrome have a 60% lifetime risk of developing breast cancer.

A. Hereditary nonpolyposis colon cancer (HNPCC), also known as Lynch syndrome, is an autosomal dominant disease that is responsible for 1% to 5% of all colon cancers. Patients with this disease have an 85% risk of developing colon cancer at some point in their lifetime. Most cancers are found within the right colon, occur at an earlier age, and are associated with better survival rates. The genetic mutation is found in a DNA mismatch repair gene that prevents replication errors. The affected genes are hMSH2 and hMLH1. No association with breast cancer has been identified with this syndrome, although women with colorectal cancers are at greater risk for developing ovarian or endometrial cancers.

C. Brown-Séquard syndrome is an incomplete spinal cord lesion clinically characterized by hemisection of the spinal cord, often in the cervical cord region. It may result from a penetrating injury to the spine or from other causes such as spinal cord tumors, degenerative disk disease, ischemia, infectious or inflammatory conditions such as meningitis, herpes simplex and zoster, tuberculosis, and syphilis. This syndrome is not associated with an increased risk for developing breast cancer.

D. Von Hippel-Lindau syndrome is an autosomal dominant, inherited, rare genetic disorder characterized by an increased risk of developing tumors. It is characterized by a predisposition to retinal angiomas, central nervous system hemangioblastomas, renal cell carcinomas, adrenal tumors, pheochromocytomas, and islet cell neoplasms of the pancreas. The CNS hemangioblastoma (Lindau tumor) is the most commonly recognized manifestation. Patients often present in the second and third decades of life, and they may present with neurologic symptoms such as headaches, ataxia, and blindness. The deficits depend on the site of the primary lesion. This syndrome is not associated with an increased risk of developing breast cancer.

E. Crow-Fukase syndrome is an extremely rare multisystem disorder that is also known as POEMS syndrome (**p**olyneuropathy, **o**rganomegaly, **e**ndocrinopathy, presence of **M**-protein, and **s**kin change). It is strongly associated with plasma cell dyscrasia. Common symptoms include progressive weakness of the nerves in the arms and legs, hepatosplenomegaly, hyperpigmentation, and hypertrichosis. Endocrine abnormalities such as failure of the gonads to function properly and diabetes mellitus type 1 may be present as well. This syndrome is not associated with an increased risk of developing breast cancer.

F. Recently described, Beckwith-Wiedemann syndrome is a rare genetic syndrome for which the cause is unclear. Approximately 80% of children with this syndrome demonstrate genotypic abnormalities of the distal region of chromosome arm 11p. This growth disorder is characterized by macrosomia, macroglossia, hemihypertrophy, visceromegaly, genital tract abnormalities, omphalocele, neonatal hypoglycemia, and embryonal tumors such as Wilms tumor, hepatoblastoma, neuroblastoma, rhabdomyosarcoma, adrenal carcinoma, and other intra-abdominal neoplasms. This syndrome is not associated with an increased risk of developing breast cancer.

38. **C.** Current guidelines for early detection of breast cancer outlined by the American Cancer Society are as follows: All women older than age 20 should perform breast self-examinations. Women 20 to 40 years of age should have a breast exam performed by a health professional every 3 years. After the age of 40, women should have an annual screening mammogram and a breast exam by a trained health professional. The National Cancer Institute guidelines recommend that women in their forties and older should have a mammogram every 1 to 2 years. Issues for obtaining mammograms for women, of all ages, are sometimes confusing and involve insurance as well as financial concerns of which practitioners should be aware. Figure 38A is the mediolateral view and Figure 38B is the craniocaudal view of normal mammography in a woman with mammographically dense breasts, which can make radiographic diagnosis in younger women difficult.

A, B, D, E. These are incorrect ages. See the guidelines outlined in the explanation for C.

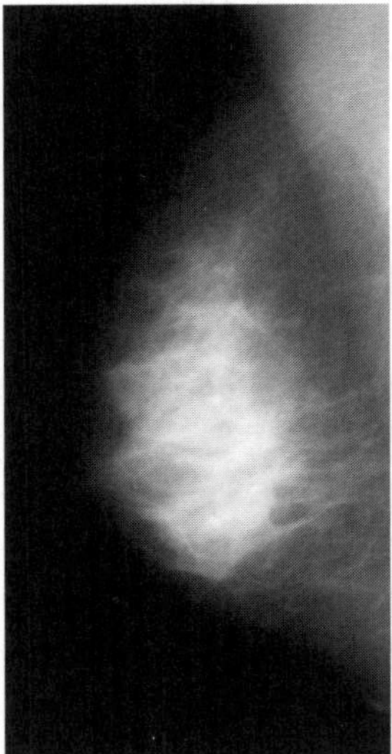

Figure 38A • Image courtesy of the University of Utah School of Medicine, Salt Lake City, Utah.

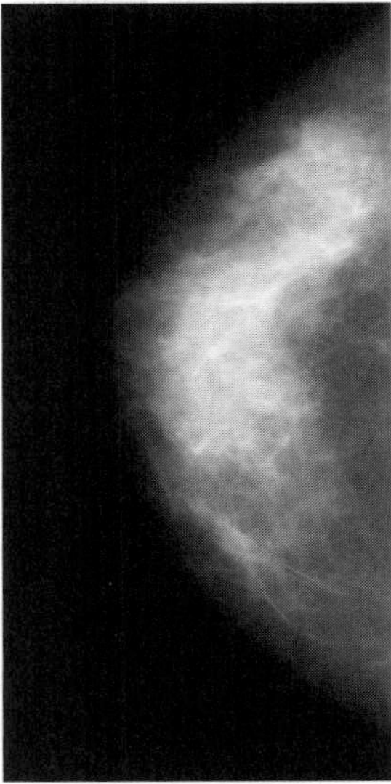

Figure 38B • Image courtesy of the University of Utah School of Medicine, Salt Lake City, Utah.

39. **D.** Lobular carcinoma in situ (LCIS) is intraepithelial proliferation of the terminal lobular-ductal unit. It does not present as a palpable mass, has no mammographic findings, and is commonly found incidentally in a breast biopsy specimen. Although LCIS is not a premalignant lesion, it is considered a marker or predictor for increased risk of breast carcinoma. Future malignancy may occur in the involved breast or in both breasts, usually in the form of infiltrative ductal carcinoma. Treatment consists mainly of close observation, as LCIS places the patient at higher risk for breast cancer. No surgical treatment is indicated at this point, even if the LCIS involves the margins of the specimen.

A, B, C, E. Because LCIS is not considered a premalignant lesion, no further treatment is warranted. The patient should be observed closely because she eventually may develop an invasive ductal or lobular carcinoma.

40. **A.** A Whipple procedure is more accurately defined as a pancreaticoduodenectomy, often done in a pyloric-preserving fashion. This procedure involves the resection of the pancreas to the level of the superior mesenteric vein, the duodenum, gallbladder, and distal common bile duct. The distal stomach and the pylorus may also need to be resected. This technically difficult operation has many potential complications, the most common of which is delayed gastric emptying. This outcome is seen in about one-third of patients.

B. Approximately 20% of patients who undergo a Whipple procedure develop a pancreatic fistula.

C. Approximately 8% of patients who undergo a Whipple procedure develop a wound infection.

D. Approximately 5% of patients who undergo a Whipple procedure develop a bile leak.

E. Approximately 5% of patients who undergo a Whipple procedure develop pancreatitis.

41. **C.** The most common type (75% to 80% of all cases) of pancreatic cancer is ductal adenocarcinoma. Pancreatic cancers occur most frequently in the head of the pancreas, 70% of the time, followed by the body (20%) and the tail (5% to 10%). Patients typically present with painless jaundice, as well as a history of anorexia and weight loss.

A, D. See the explanation for C.

B, E. These terms are not normally associated with anatomical areas of the pancreas.

42. **B.** The primary diagnostic maneuver in any patient with a suspicious neck mass is to obtain a fine-needle aspiration (FNA); indeed, this procedure is considered the gold standard for evaluation of a thyroid nodule. The false-negative rate for FNA is less than 5%, and the false-positive rate is less than 2%. The FNA can be performed in an office or clinic setting with minimal discomfort and expense to the patient. If the mass is small or indistinct, ultrasound guidance can be used during the FNA. When positive findings occur, treatment can proceed without further delay. If the FNA result is negative, further diagnostic procedures should be performed.

A. Obtaining a CT of the neck may be an appropriate step, but it should occur following an FNA result.

C. An incisional biopsy is hardly ever performed, especially in a mass of this size, because it may leave involved tissue behind.

D. A lobectomy may eventually be required to obtain a diagnostic result or to treat the mass, but a less invasive means of diagnosis should be attempted initially.

E. Thyroidectomy is not indicated as an initial diagnostic test.

43. **E.** Papillary thyroid carcinoma is the most common form of thyroid cancer. It is associated with prior exposure to ionizing radiation, has a propensity for local or regional recurrence, and usually spreads via lymphatics. Nearly 50% of patients will have spread to regional lymph nodes at the time of diagnosis. Treatment consists of surgical excision, with the extent of excision being a topic of considerable controversy. Physicians at the M. D. Anderson Cancer Center advocate total thyroidectomy for papillary tumors larger than 1 cm. This procedure is combined with a neck dissection if clinically palpable nodes are present. Total thyroidectomy allows for postoperative radio-iodine ablation, which has been shown to decrease local–regional relapse rates by as much as 50%. Thymoglobulin may also be used as part of monitoring for recurrent disease.

A. Enucleation is inappropriate as it carries the risks of hemorrhage, recurrent laryngeal nerve injury, and incomplete exam of the tumor.

B. A lobectomy is used as a diagnostic measure in thyroid nodules with an unclear diagnosis. In papillary carcinoma, there is no role for lobectomy alone.

C. A lobectomy with isthmectomy is a reasonable treatment for a papillary carcinoma less than 1 cm in size.

D. Subtotal thyroidectomy is reserved for noncancer thyroid surgery, mainly debulking of a large goiter. Currently, many surgeons would advocate for a complete thyroidectomy with thyroid hormone replacement as surgical treatment for the lesion described.

44. **D.** Most thyroid carcinomas recur within 5 years of initial treatment. Thyroglobulin values normally drop after thyroidectomy and ablation and, as such, serve as a sensitive indicator of recurrent or persistent disease.

A, B, E. TSH, free T_4, and T_3 reuptake levels will depend on the adequacy of thyroid replacement. These three levels will not indicate whether recurrent disease is present.

C. Calcitonin is analyzed as part of screening for medullary thyroid cancer, not papillary thyroid cancer.

45. **A.** *Helicobacter pylori* infection, one of the most common human bacterial infectious diseases, is causally linked to gastritis, gastric ulcers, peptic ulcer disease, gastric adenocarcinoma, and gastric B-cell lymphoma. *H. pylori* is a gram-negative spiral organism that is both slow growing and highly motile. Approximately 70% to 90% of patients with duodenal ulcers have concomitant *H. pylori* infections. In the case of gastric ulcers, 50% to 70% will be associated with an *H. pylori* infection. It is believed that such an infection may disrupt the protective mucosal layers, thereby predisposing the patient to ulcer development. Treatment of the *H. pylori* infection will increase healing of the ulcers and decrease the rate of recurrence.

B. *H. pylori* infection has been implicated in the development of gastric lymphoma, but not to the same degree that it is associated with gastric or duodenal ulcers. It may be linked to as many as 40% of tumors in communities with a low incidence of gastric lymphomas.

C. Esophageal ulcers are most commonly caused by GERD, drug ingestion, and caustic injuries. The relationship between *H. pylori* and GERD is controversial and involves the prevalence and protective treatment for *H. pylori* in GERD patients.

D. The incidence of gastric carcinoma and *H. pylori* infection is similar to the incidence of gastric lymphoma and *H. pylori* infection.

E. Chronic use of NSAIDs increases the risk of ulcer disease but not in association with *H. pylori* infection.

F. Mucosa-associated lymphoid tissue lymphoma (MALToma) is an *H. pylori*–related tumor of B-cell origin. Evidence suggests that a significant proportion of primary gastrointestinal lymphomas are driven by exogenous agents/antigens. In the stomach, *H. pylori* appears to be responsible for most cases of low-grade lymphomas (MALToma).

46. **A.** Treatment with bismuth subsalicylate and metronidazole is the least costly initial treatment for *H. pylori* infection.

B. A parietal cell vagotomy is not indicated unless complications of peptic ulcer disease occur.

C. Proton pump inhibitors are not indicated as treatment for *H. pylori* infection and may obscure test results for the presence of *H. pylori*.

D. H_2 blockers will decrease acid levels but will not treat the infecting organism.

E. Mucosal barrier drugs, such as sucralfate, may protect the mucosa but will not eradicate the *H. pylori* organism.

47. **D.** This patient's history is very concerning for an esophageal mass. Symptoms of a mass include unwanted weight loss and dysphagia, which initially is to solids but progresses to liquids. Risk factors include tobacco and alcohol use, male gender, African American ethnicity, nitrosamine ingestion, and history of gastroesophageal reflux disease. Although all of these examination choices may eventually be obtained in the total work-up for esophageal carcinoma, endoscopic evaluation provides the most information and allows tissue samples to be obtained for pathology. Endoscopic ultrasound can also be performed, providing information regarding clinical stage.

A, B. Although a mass in the esophagus may be identified via upper GI imaging or esophagram, an endoscopy will provide even more information because of the access to the mass for biopsy.

C. A thoracic CT will eventually be needed to assist in the staging of an esophageal mass, but it is not the first choice in evaluation.

E. An enteroclysis is a fluoroscopic contrast study of the small bowel. Examination of the esophagus is not part of this study.

48. **E.** Acute rejection—a cellular-mediated response—is a result of sensitized lymphocytes and may occur days to weeks following transplantation. The pathology of a kidney biopsy reveals graft infiltration of small lymphocytes and mononuclear cells. High-dose steroids or antilymphocyte medications can usually reverse acute rejection.

A, C. These options describe chronic rejection. This condition usually occurs months to years following transplantation and is due to both cellular and humoral immune responses. The antigens responsible are usually the minor histocompatibility antigens. Unfortunately, this type of rejection is currently irreversible.

B, D. These descriptions refer to hyperacute rejection, which occurs when the recipient has preformed antibodies, which should be discovered in pretransplant cross matching of donor lymphocytes with recipient serum. It begins immediately after revascularization of the graft secondary to neutrophil infiltration and complement-mediated injury to the vascular endothelium. Treatment consists of graft removal.

49. **A.** A post-transplant lymphocele occurs in approximately 15% of renal transplant cases. It is caused by inadequate ligation of lymphatics transected along the iliac vessels or lymph leakage from the allograft. Diagnosis is made by needle aspiration of the fluid collection and by obtaining culture and chemistry analyses of the aspirate. Large fluid collections may compromise renal function due to the compression of the kidney, ureter, or bladder. Recurrent lymphoceles may be treated by repeated aspiration, but multiple aspirations, pose a significant risk of infection. Better long-term solutions include intraperitoneal drainage by removing the lymphocele wall. Omentoplasty is also done to decrease the likelihood of recurrence. This procedure may be performed laparoscopically or via laparotomy, depending on factors such as location and size of the fluid collection. The US image (see Figure 49) shows the large fluid collection adjacent to the kidney, consistent with a lymphocele.

B. From the information presented, there is no indication of nephrotoxicity from Prograf.

C, D. These choices are appropriate if fluid aspiration of the lymphocele does not lead to improved renal function.

E. Because renal function is already compromised, further observation is not appropriate.

50. **C.** This patient has reactivation of herpes zoster, or shingles. This condition affects approximately 30% of transplant patients, usually arising within the first 6 months after transplantation. Treatment initially consists of IV acyclovir followed by an oral course of the same therapy. This treatment helps to prevent systemic dissemination and aids in healing of the skin lesions. Immunosuppression should also be reduced to aid in recovery, an approach that also reduces mortality. In patients with systemic disseminated disease, hyperimmune globulin may be administered as well. Affected patients should undergo a bronchoscopy to rule out superinfection of the lungs.

A. A more aggressive approach than oral acyclovir should be taken to prevent systemic dissemination, which is associated with a higher mortality rate.

B. A reduction of immunosuppressive medication is only part of the appropriate treatment regimen.

D. Increasing immunosuppressive medications may actually intensify the current infection.

E. Observation alone is not appropriate for this situation.

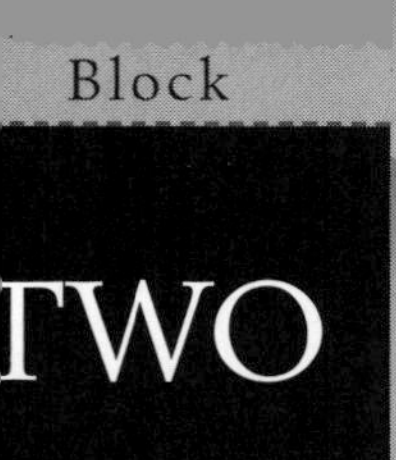

Block

TWO Questions

Setting 2: Office

Your office is in a primary care generalist group practice located in a physician office suite adjoining a suburban community hospital. Patients are usually seen by appointment. Most of the patients you see are from your own practice and are appearing for regular scheduled return visits, with some new patients as well. As in most group practices, you will often encounter a patient whose primary care is managed by one of your associates; reference may be made to the patient's medical records. You may do some telephone management, and you may have to respond to questions about articles in magazines and on television that will require interpretation. Complete laboratory and radiology services are available.

The next two questions (items 51 and 52) correspond to the following vignette.

A 47-year-old male is seen in your office complaining of left scrotal swelling. The patient states that he first noticed the swelling more than a month ago, while showering. The patient denies dysuria or penile discharge, but over the last 4 months he has inadvertently lost 15 pounds. On examination, you identify the swelling as a varicocele.

51. In this clinical situation, what should you consider as an etiology of this problem?

A. Testicular cancer
B. Inguinal hernia
C. Renal cell carcinoma
D. Epididymitis
E. Testicular torsion

52. The left testicular vein most commonly drains into which of the following structures?

A. Renal vein
B. Inferior vena cava
C. Inferior adrenal vein
D. Internal iliac vein
E. Common testicular vein

End of set

The next three questions (items 53–55) correspond to the following vignette.

A 32-year-old male presents to your office with concerns about a new mole on his right shoulder. The patient's wife was the first to notice it about 2 weeks ago. The patient reports that he has smoked one pack of cigarettes per day for the last 5 years. History also includes frequent sunburns when he worked as a lifeguard while in high school, with present employment as a salesman. Family medical history is unremarkable with the exception that his father is treated for hypertension. On exam, you note an irregular, pigmented lesion approximately 7 mm in diameter. There are no palpable lymph nodes. You perform an excision of the lesion in the office and send it to pathology.

53. What risk factor is most significant for disease in the patient's history?

A. Age
B. Smoking history
C. Previous surgery
D. History of severe sunburn
E. Fair skin

54. The pathology results are consistent with a 1.2 mm deep melanoma with clear margins. What is the most important prognostic determinant?

A. Width of the lesion
B. Patient age
C. Depth of the lesion
D. Location of the lesion
E. Color of the lesion

55. What should the surgical margin of this patient's excised melanoma be?

A. 0.5 cm
B. 1 cm
C. 2 cm
D. 3 cm
E. 4 cm

End of set

The next four questions (items 56–59) correspond to the following vignette.

A 25-year-old male was diagnosed with a pheochromocytoma 6 months ago. The patient underwent a successful adrenalectomy and returns to your office for a follow-up appointment. His physical exam is normal except for a palpable thyroid mass. Lab values obtained reveal a serum calcium level of 11.5 mg/dL.

56. Multiple endocrine neoplasia (MEN) type IIa syndrome is associated with pheochromocytoma, medullary thyroid cancer, and which of the following?

A. Neurofibromas
B. Marfanoid habitus
C. Insulinoma
D. Pituitary tumor
E. Parathyroid hyperplasia

57. What is the best way to screen for medullary thyroid cancer?

A. Serum calcitonin
B. TSH levels
C. Serum calcium
D. Frequent ultrasounds
E. Random fine-needle aspirations

58. This patient's MEN type II syndrome is associated with which of the following genes?

A. p53
B. ras
C. RET
D. bcl
E. n-myc

59. Where are the inferior parathyroid glands embryologically derived?

A. First pharyngeal pouch
B. Second pharyngeal pouch
C. Third pharyngeal pouch
D. Fourth pharyngeal pouch
E. Fifth pharyngeal pouch

End of set

The next two questions (items 60 and 61) correspond to the following vignette.

A 28-year-old female who recently underwent a laparoscopic appendectomy for appendicitis presents to your office for evaluation of a 12 cm liver mass that was incidentally found on a CT scan (Figure 60) obtained prior to appendectomy. The patient is otherwise very healthy with no significant medical or surgical history. Medications taken include oral contraceptive pills and acetaminophen for occasional headaches.

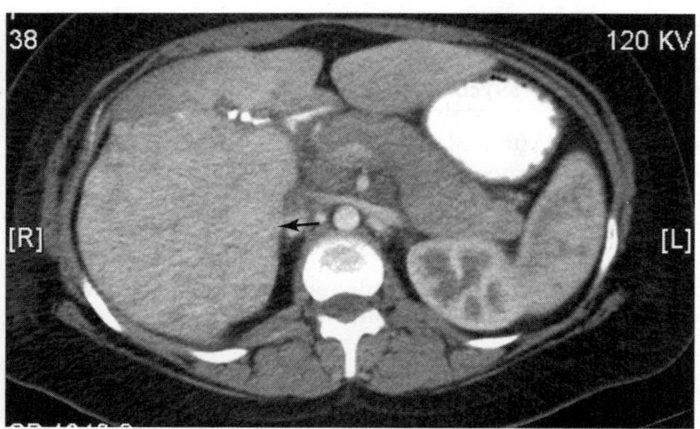

Figure 60 • Image courtesy of the University of Utah School of Medicine, Salt Lake City, Utah.

60. What do you suspect this lesion to most likely be?

A. Hepatoma
B. Hepatic adenoma
C. Focal nodular hyperplasia
D. Hemangioendothelioma
E. Hemangioma

61. Which of the following is true regarding this patient's lesion and proper management?

A. Carries a 60% chance of malignant degeneration
B. Carries a risk of spontaneous rupture and bleeding
C. Will regress with cessation of the inciting agent
D. Caused by chronic use of acetaminophen
E. Often found to have distant metastases

End of set

62. A 31-year-old female presents to your office with a history of a pigmented lesion on her shoulder. Recently the lesion has become significantly darker and increasingly irregular in shape. You perform an excisional biopsy, and the pathology comes back as a 0.9 mm deep Clarks II melanoma. What is the most common type of melanoma?

A. Lentigo maligna melanoma
B. Superficial spreading melanoma
C. Acral lentiginous melanoma
D. Nodular melanoma
E. Ocular melanoma

The next three questions (items 63–65) correspond to the following vignette:

A 46-year-old female presents to your office and reports a 6-month history of palpitations, diaphoresis, tremulousness, irritability, and weakness. The patient notices the symptoms most frequently after having not eaten for several hours. You suspect she may have an endocrine tumor.

63. Which type of neuroendocrine tumor is most likely associated with this patient's presentation?

A. Carcinoid
B. Gastrinoma
C. Insulinoma
D. Glucagonoma
E. Somatostatinoma

64. What is the most appropriate diagnostic step in the work-up of this patient?

A. CT scan of the abdomen
B. Ultrasound of the abdomen
C. Euglycemic C-peptide suppression test
D. 72-hour fast with measurement of glucose, insulin, and C-peptide levels
E. Trial course of diazoxide

65. Which triad of symptoms is suggestive of this diagnosis?

A. Beck's triad
B. Whipple's triad
C. Charcot's triad
D. Virchow's triad
E. Ostlund's triad

End of set

The next three questions (items 66–68) correspond to the following vignette.

A mother brings her otherwise healthy 11-month-old male child to your office for evaluation of an abdominal mass the mother first noticed 2 weeks ago while at the swimming pool. The mass has not changed in size and does not seem to bother the child. The child has not experienced any vomiting and his bowel function is unchanged. You suspect the child has a neuroblastoma.

66. What is the most likely location site of childhood neuroblastoma?

- **A.** Neck
- **B.** Mediastinum
- **C.** Adrenal gland
- **D.** Spleen
- **E.** Pelvis

67. You take this infant to the operating room and excise the neuroblastoma. The child does well through surgery and recovery, and the tumor is pathologically determined to fit the Stage I classification. Which of the following are factors used to determine stage in childhood neuroblastoma?

- **A.** Nodal status and tumor crossing the midline
- **B.** Tumor response to preoperative chemo-radiation
- **C.** Amplification of the c-myc gene
- **D.** Primary anatomical site
- **E.** Frequency of constitutional symptoms

68. Amplification of which oncogene is associated with a neuroblastoma?

- **A.** k-ras
- **B.** n-myc
- **C.** c-abl
- **D.** HER-2/neu
- **E.** c-myc

End of set

The next three questions (items 69–71) correspond to the following vignette.

A 52-year-old female presents to your office for evaluation of a 3-day history of abdominal pain. Medical-surgical history includes a total abdominal hysterectomy with bilateral salpingo-oophorectomy 3 years ago, at which time she was found to have an ovarian mass. The mass was a serous cystadenocarcinoma, limited to the ovary. During the last 3 days the patient's pain has worsened, and she also complains of feeling bloated. In the last 12 hours she has experienced three episodes of bilious emesis. Her last bowel movement was 2 days ago, and she reports having flatus approximately 2 hours ago. Vital signs are as follows: BP 142/78, HR 98, RR 16, T 38.1°C. All labs are normal. You obtain an abdominal film (Figure 69).

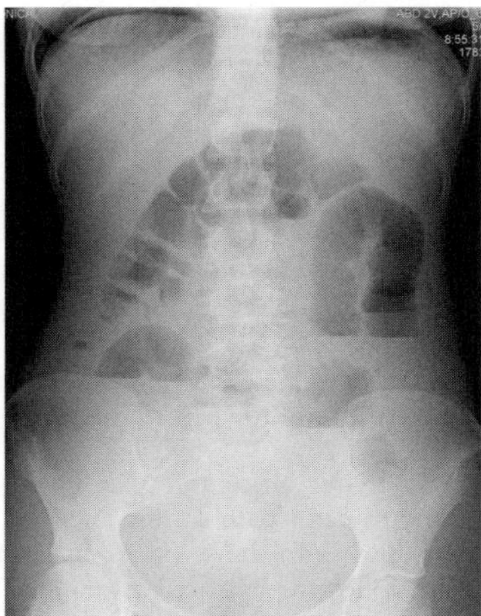

Figure 69 • Image courtesy of the University of Utah School of Medicine, Salt Lake City, Utah.

69. What is the most likely cause of this patient's abdominal pain?

- A. Primary small bowel tumor
- B. Metastatic ovarian cancer to the small bowel
- C. Adhesive band
- D. Internal hernia
- E. Ileus

70. Which of the following statements is most appropriate relative to the initial medical management of this patient's disorder?

- A. Bowel rest with immediate use of TPN is recommended.
- B. NGT decompression has no role in modern SBO management.
- C. IV antibiotics should always be given.
- D. Placement of a Foley catheter, NGT, and fluid resuscitation are standard measures.
- E. Medical management of SBO is never indicated.

71. You decide to admit the patient to the hospital. After starting your initial therapy, she feels somewhat better. Over the next few days there continues to be high output from the NGT. On hospital day 4, the patient's abdomen remains distended and she develops focal tenderness in the right lower quadrant. The CBC shows a WBC count of 15,400 and the patient's temperature is 38.7°C with a heart rate of 113. What is the most appropriate next step in this patient's management?

- A. Three-view image of the abdomen
- B. Enteroclysis
- C. CT scan of the abdomen
- D. Upper endoscopy
- E. Emergent exploratory laparotomy

End of set

72. A 72-year-old male with a 45-pack-per-year history of smoking comes to your office complaining of blood in his urine. You work up the hematuria and diagnose the patient with a transitional cell carcinoma of the bladder. Based on your preoperative work-up, you believe this to be a T1 tumor. What is the proper management of this tumor?

- A. Local radiation therapy
- B. Chemotherapy
- C. Chemotherapy and radiation therapy
- D. Transurethral resection with chemotherapy
- E. Radical cystectomy with radiation and chemotherapy

The next two questions (items 73 and 74) correspond to the following vignette.

A 35-year-old male who is a known narcotic abuser visits your office complaining of abdominal pain. The patient is unable to sit still and writhes in pain during the examination. The pain is mainly in the right flank, travels down into the scrotum, began today around 5 P.M., and has progressively worsened. The following labs were obtained: WBC 8000, BUN 15 mg/dL, creatinine 1.0 mg/dL, and UA demonstrated microscopic hematuria. A CT scan is obtained (Figure 73A).

73. What is the most appropriate next step in the treatment of this patient?

- A. Emergent ureteroscopy
- B. Narcotics for pain
- C. Exploratory laparotomy
- D. Nonsteroidal anti-inflammatory drugs for pain
- E. No treatment; the patient is seeking narcotics

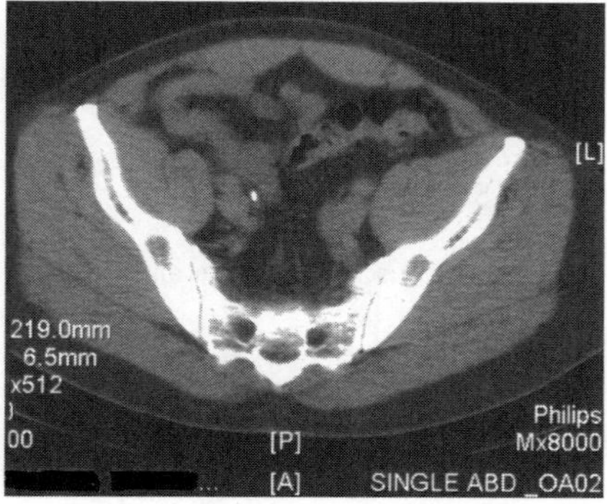

Figure 73A • Image courtesy of the University of Utah School of Medicine, Salt Lake City, Utah.

74. What type of renal calculi is most commonly encountered in patients who have undergone small bowel bypass surgery?

- A. Uric acid
- B. Calcium oxalate
- C. Cystine
- D. Struvite
- E. Cysteine

End of set

The next two questions (items 75 and 76) correspond to the following vignette.

A 51-year-old, previously healthy male presents to your office for evaluation of a gastric carcinoma that was found on an upper endoscopy performed for persistent emesis associated with anemia and a 20-pound weight loss over the last 3 months. The tumor is located in the gastric cardia. CT evaluation shows some enlarged perigastric lymph nodes, but no evidence of distant metastasis.

75. Which of the following factors is associated with an increased risk for developing adenocarcinoma of the stomach?

A. High-fat diet
B. Smoked foods
C. Chewing tobacco
D. Japanese ancestry
E. Diet high in fruits and vegetables

76. Which of the following statements best describes the location of gastric tumors?

A. The distribution is evenly split between the antrum and the body of the stomach.
B. Tumors rarely occupy the entire stomach.
C. The distribution is evenly split between the antrum, the body, and the cardia of the stomach.
D. The distribution is evenly split between the cardia and the body of the stomach.
E. The distribution is evenly split between the antrum and the corpus.
F. There is no pattern to gastric tumor location.

End of set

The next two questions (items 77 and 78) correspond to the following vignette.

A 75-year-old male visits your office complaining of fatigue and dizziness. The patient has been feeling much better during the last 2 days, but earlier this morning had a large bowel movement with gross blood. Vital signs have remained stable: BP 119/82, HR 92, T 37.2°C, and SaO_2 95% on room air. Presently, the patient is alert and the physical exam is unremarkable. Rectal exam shows a moderate amount of gross blood. The following labs are obtained: WBC 7000, HCT 34%, PLT 130,000, Na 141 mmol/L, K 4.1 mmol/L, Cl 108 mmol/L, BUN 35 mg/dL, creatinine 1.0 mg/dL, and glucose 120 mg/dL.

77. What is the most appropriate first step in management of this patient?

A. Diagnostic laparoscopy
B. CT scan
C. Colonoscopy
D. Angiography
E. Exploratory laparotomy

78. What is the most common cause of this patient's lower GI bleeding?

A. Ulcerative colitis
B. Colon cancer
C. Meckel's diverticulum
D. Vascular ectasia
E. Diverticulosis

End of set

The next three questions (items 79–81) correspond to the following vignette.

An 18-year-old female is referred to your office by a local hematologist. The patient was diagnosed 6 weeks ago with autoimmune hemolytic anemia. Since then she has been repeatedly treated with glucocorticoids, but continues to require blood transfusions. After discussing the options with the patient's parents, they elect to pursue a splenectomy.

79. To perform the splenectomy, you must know your anatomy. The splenic vein empties into which of the following?

A. Inferior mesenteric vein
B. Superior mesenteric vein
C. Inferior vena cava
D. Azygous vein
E. Portal vein

80. When considering splenectomy, this patient will require which of the following?

A. Vaccinations for encapsulated organisms
B. Preoperative CT scan to evaluate splenic size
C. Type and cross for platelet transfusion
D. An open splenectomy to evaluate for accessory spleens intraoperatively
E. Routine LUQ drains

81. The patient does well postoperatively and is discharged from the hospital on postoperative day 5. On the return visit to your clinic, you check the patient's CBC and find a stable hematocrit at 36% with a platelet count of 1,400,000. What is the most appropriate next step in her management?

A. Aspirin
B. Heparin drip
C. Coumadin
D. Lovenox
E. No treatment needed

End of set

The next three questions (items 82–84) correspond to the following vignette.

A 68-year-old female visits your office with complaints of constipation for many years, sometimes to the point of self-digitalization. Most recently, the patient experienced the onset of rectal pain along with blood and mucous discharge each time she has a bowel movement. On physical examination, the anus and anoderm are normal but the patient has severe tenesmus.

82. What is the most likely cause of her perirectal pain?

- **A.** Perirectal abscess with spontaneous drainage
- **B.** Rectal polyp or cancer
- **C.** Anal fissure
- **D.** Solitary rectal ulcer
- **E.** Anal condylomata

83. What is the best initial therapy for this patient?

- **A.** Stool softeners, bulking agents, and bowel retraining
- **B.** Narcotic pain medication with close follow-up
- **C.** Surgical closure
- **D.** Exam under anesthesia
- **E.** Topical nitroglycerin

84. The patient follows this treatment for several weeks, but returns to your office with complaints of persistent pain and minimal improvement in her condition. What is the next step in management of this patient?

- **A.** A trial of sucralfate enemas for 6 weeks
- **B.** Abdominoperineal resection
- **C.** Internal anal sphincterotomy
- **D.** Low anterior resection
- **E.** Diverting colostomy

End of set

The next three questions (items 85–87) correspond to the following vignette.

A 65-year-old male returns to your office for his annual physical examination. The patient reports that his general state of good health has continued, that he has not been hospitalized recently, and that he has continued to take atorvastatin and aspirin on a daily basis. Laboratory values from a year ago were unremarkable. Physical exam today is unremarkable except for a firm, irregular area felt on his prostate during a digital rectal exam. Laboratory values are as follows: WBC 8000, HCT 42%, PLT 148,000, Na 142 mmol/L, K 3.9 mmol/L, Cl 110 mmol/L, HCO_3 24 mmol/L, BUN 15 mg/dL, creatinine 1.1 mg/dL, glucose 110 mg/dL, Ca 11 mg/dL, alkaline phosphate 112 U/L, PSA 10 ng/mL, total bilirubin 0.8 mg/dL, AST 12 U/L, and ALT 25 U/L.

85. What is the most appropriate initial step in the management of this patient?

- **A.** Cystoscopy with washings
- **B.** Transrectal ultrasound with biopsy
- **C.** Pelvic CT scan
- **D.** Observation
- **E.** Pelvic MRI

86. After further evaluation, the patient is found to have stage B1 prostate cancer (a 1.3 cm nodule in the peripheral zone of the prostate). What is the standard treatment for this patient's stage of prostate cancer?

- **A.** Observation
- **B.** External beam radiation
- **C.** Total prostatectomy with pelvic lymphadenectomy
- **D.** Hormonal therapy alone
- **E.** Repeat pelvic MRI

87. A year later the patient returns to your office for routine follow-up. The patient states that he has been doing relatively well, although he complains of some general malaise as well as body aches. Vital signs are within normal limits, and the physical exam is unrevealing. Laboratory values are as follows: WBC 5000, HCT 40%, PLT 152,000, Na 140 mmol/L, K 3.5 mmol/L, Cl 109 mmol/L, HCO_3 24 mmol/L, BUN 12 mg/dL, creatinine 1.0 mg/dL, glucose 91 mg/dL, Ca 10.5 mg/dL, alkaline phosphate 365 U/L, PSA 8 ng/mL, total bilirubin 0.9 mg/dL, AST 21 U/L, and ALT 22 U/L. Which of the following most likely accounts for these findings?

- **A.** Sarcoidosis
- **B.** Osteoclastic bone metastasis
- **C.** Cholestasis
- **D.** Osteoblastic bone metastasis
- **E.** Vitamin D deficiency

End of set

The next three questions (items 88–90) correspond to the following vignette.

An 11-year-old male is seen in your office for complaints of left knee pain. Both the patient and his mother tell you that the pain has been present for the last 6 months but has progressively become more severe. The pain is more intense in the evening and usually prevents the patient from sleeping. The child denies any trauma and, according to his mother, is otherwise healthy without any other medical problems. Past history does not include any surgery, and the child is not taking any medications. Currently he attends sixth grade at the local elementary school, where he is an excellent student. Physical exam shows a large, tender mass fixed to the posteromedial distal femur, a knee that is somewhat flexed, and severe pain produced upon passive range of motion.

88. What is the most likely diagnosis?

   A. Osteoclastoma
   B. Ewing's sarcoma
   C. Chondrosarcoma
   D. Unicameral bone cyst
   E. Osteogenic sarcoma

89. What is a common historical finding in a patient with this disease?

   A. Multiple, small skin tumors
   B. Premature birth
   C. History of loose, bloody stools
   D. Prior broken bones
   E. A history of retinoblastoma as an infant

90. What is the most appropriate treatment for this patient's mass?

   A. Neoadjuvant chemotherapy, limb-sparing surgery, and adjuvant chemotherapy
   B. Radiation with delayed amputation
   C. Radiation therapy followed by tumor excision
   D. Amputation and systemic chemotherapy
   E. Limb amputation

End of set

The next five questions (items 91–95) correspond to the following vignette.

A 48-year-old female member of your staff has been enjoying brownies at the office holiday party when she experiences an acute onset of abdominal pain. The patient states that her pain is primarily in the right upper quadrant, is persistent in nature, and radiates to the subscapular area. The patient has not experienced similar pain in the past. Her abdomen is diffusely tender and rigid on exam. Laboratory values are as follows: WBC 13,000, HCT 39%, PLT 213,000, Na 140 mmol/L, K 3.8 mmol/L, Cl 105 mmol/L, HCO_3 23 mmol/L, BUN 12 mg/dL, creatinine 1.1 mg/dL, glucose 100 mg/dL, amylase 250 U/L, and lipase 35 U/L. A previous right upper quadrant ultrasound, obtained 6 months ago, shows no evidence of stones within the gallbladder or ductal dilatation.

91. What is the next step in this patient's management?

- **A.** Repeat an abdominal ultrasound
- **B.** Increase the pain medication
- **C.** CT scan of the abdomen
- **D.** Emergent surgery
- **E.** Fluid bolus

92. The appropriate management is performed, and the patient is found to have a perforated prepyloric gastric ulcer. Which type of gastric ulcer is this?

- **A.** Type I
- **B.** Type II
- **C.** Type III
- **D.** Type IV
- **E.** Type V

93. The patient is extremely concerned and wants to know more about the procedure you performed. You counsel her that which of the following is the most appropriate surgical procedure?

- **A.** Vagotomy and pyloroplasty
- **B.** Total gastrectomy
- **C.** Highly selective vagotomy
- **D.** Distal gastrectomy, which includes the ulcer with a Billroth II gastrojejunostomy
- **E.** Vagotomy and gastrojejunostomy
- **F.** Proximal gastric resection, which includes the ulcer

94. The patient has an uncomplicated hospital stay and is discharged on postoperative day 5. Two weeks later she returns to your office for follow-up. The patient complains of distention and nausea following meals associated with right upper quadrant pain that is relieved by vomiting. This problem consistently occurs with meals. The patient denies fever or chills, and the abdominal exam shows a well healed wound. What is the most likely cause of the patient's symptoms?

- **A.** Recurrent ulcer
- **B.** Postprandial dumping syndrome
- **C.** Afferent loop syndrome
- **D.** Postvagotomy diarrhea
- **E.** Bile reflux gastritis

95. Which condition following this patient's procedure is associated with abdominal pain and fullness, vomiting, diarrhea, flushing, palpitations, and dizziness?

A. Recurrent ulcer
B. Early postprandial dumping syndrome
C. Afferent loop syndrome
D. Late postprandial dumping syndrome
E. Bile reflux gastritis

End of set

The next two questions (items 96 and 97) correspond to the following vignette.

An 8-year-old female is referred to your office for evaluation of recurrent abdominal pain. The child describes the pain as occurring periodically and not associated with eating. The child's mother notes that her eyes occasionally will appear somewhat yellow. On physical exam, you are able to reproduce some discomfort with deep palpation and you detect a slight fullness in the right upper quadrant. There is no evidence of peritonitis. Past medical history is significant for a similar episode of pain with a slight fever and jaundice approximately 10 months ago, but the patient has otherwise been healthy.

96. You are concerned this patient may have what condition?

A. Acute cholecystitis
B. Acute cholangitis
C. Pancreatic head mass
D. Choledochal cyst
E. Choledocholithiasis

97. What is the most appropriate initial diagnostic study in this child?

A. Right upper quadrant ultrasound
B. Abdominal CT scan
C. Hepatobiliary scintigraphy
D. Endoscopic retrograde cholangiopancreatography
E. Percutaneous transhepatic cholangiography

End of set

The next three questions (items 98–100) correspond to the following vignette.

A 67-year-old male with a history of alcoholic cirrhosis is referred to your clinic for evaluation of a liver mass found on a CT scan. The patient has been complaining to his wife of vague, right upper quadrant pain and has lost 20 pounds during the last 4 months. The patient has been previously diagnosed with Child's class A cirrhosis. History includes well-controlled hypertension and a coronary artery bypass graft (CABG) performed 3 years ago. The patient has a 44-pack-per-year history of smoking and quit 3 years ago, after his CABG. Surgical history includes an open appendectomy at age 9.

98. What is the most likely type of mass in this patient's liver?

- **A.** Hepatocellular carcinoma
- **B.** Cholangiocarcinoma
- **C.** Hepatoblastoma
- **D.** Hemangioma
- **E.** Adenoma

99. Which tumor marker is most often associated with this type of tumor?

- **A.** β-hCG
- **B.** α-fetoprotein
- **C.** CA 19-9
- **D.** Carcinoembryonic antigen
- **E.** CA 125

100. What is the most common site of distant metastasis of this type of tumor?

- **A.** Brain
- **B.** Spleen
- **C.** Small bowel
- **D.** Pancreas
- **E.** Lungs

End of set

Block

TWO Answers and Explanations

Block

TWO

Answer Key

51. C
52. A
53. D
54. C
55. C
56. E
57. A
58. C
59. C
60. B
61. B
62. B
63. C
64. D
65. B
66. C
67. A
68. B
69. C
70. D
71. E
72. D
73. B
74. B
75. B
76. C
77. C
78. E
79. E
80. A
81. A
82. D
83. A
84. A
85. B
86. C
87. D
88. E
89. E
90. A
91. D
92. C
93. D
94. C
95. B
96. D
97. A
98. A
99. B
100. E

51. **C.** Renal cell carcinoma (RCC) causes 2% of cancer deaths. It is seen in males twice as often as in females. The classic clinical triad consists of flank pain, hematuria, and a palpable abdominal mass; however, it is seen in only 10% to 15 % of cases. The abdominal CT scan (Figure 51) shows a large, left renal mass (note arrows).

A. Every testicular mass should be investigated with suspicion of testicular cancer and should be included in this patient's differential diagnosis. However, testicular cancer usually presents as a solid, painless testicular mass rather than as a soft venous collection above the testis.

B. An inguinal hernia should be considered, but can usually be ruled out by physical exam.

D. Epididymitis also includes a painful, swollen mass in the scrotum relieved by elevation and antibiotics.

E. Testicular torsion involves a very painful, swollen testis.

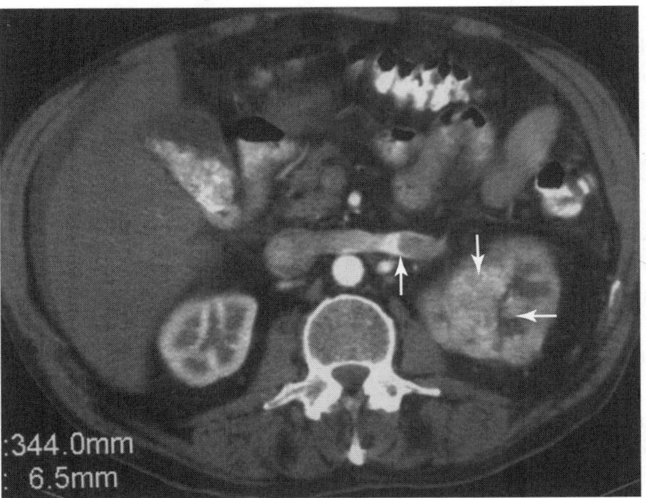

Figure 51 • Image courtesy of the University of Utah School of Medicine, Salt Lake City, Utah.

52. **A.** In RCC, the renal vein should be thoroughly investigated, as tumor thrombus may spread into the lumen of the inferior vena cava (IVC). Figure 51 demonstrates RCC of the left kidney with probable tumor extension into the left renal vein (note arrows). Because the left testicular vein drains into the left renal vein, IVC involvement may lead to increased pressure within the left testicular vein commonly seen as testicular varicosities, also known as varicoceles.

B. The right testicular vein will drain into the inferior vena cava.

C. The left inferior adrenal vein usually drains into the left renal vein.

D. The internal iliac vein drains the pelvis but not the testes.

E. There is no common testicular vein.

53. **D.** The incidence of melanoma has tripled in the last three decades and currently affects 5 to 25 per 100,000 people. Risk factors include severe sunburn before age 18, giant congenital nevus syndrome, family history of melanoma, multiple dysplastic nevi syndrome, and Caucasian race. Early detection significantly improves the results of treatment. Clinically suspicious lesions include those that change in size or color, itch, ulcerate, or bleed. Work as a lifeguard in high school would suggest significant sun exposure.

A. Age is a relative risk factor, but not as significant as sun exposure.

B. Smoking history is a relative risk factor, but not as significant as sun exposure.

C. Prior surgery is not a risk factor, unless the procedure was to remove a previous melanoma.

E. Although fair skin is considered a risk factor, it does not correlate with melanoma incidence as much as a history of early severe sun exposure or burns.

54. **C.** Tumor depth is the most accurate index of metastatic potential. Breslow's classification of staging is determined by tumor thickness as measured by pathologists: 1.0 mm or less, 1.01 to 2.00 mm, 2.01 to 4.00 mm, and greater than 4.00 mm. The greater the depth involved, the higher the risk of regional and distant metastasis as well as local recurrence.

A. Although the width of the lesion may make obtaining clear margins difficult, as with facial lesions, it is the depth of the lesion that determines prognosis.

B. Age contributes little to the overall prognosis with melanoma.

D. In terms of location, acral lentiginous melanoma usually occurs on the palms, soles, and under the nails. This type is the most aggressive form of melanoma. Tumor depth still is the most important information for prognosis.

E. The color of the lesion has no effect on prognosis.

55. **C.** A full-thickness excisional biopsy is the preferred treatment. The depth of invasion determines the size of the surgical margin. Lesions less than 1 mm thick require 1 cm margins. A surgical margin of 2 cm is adequate for lesions greater than 1 mm thick. There has been much debate in the literature concerning the surgical margin for melanoma. The minimum margin for intermediate-thickness melanoma (1 to 4 mm) is 2 cm. For tumor depths greater than 4 mm, the adequate margin size is 2 to 3 cm.

A, B, D, E. See the explanation for C.

56. **E.** Multiple endocrine neoplasia (MEN) type II syndrome is also known as Sipple's syndrome. It is typically classified as one of two types. Type IIa consists of medullary thyroid carcinoma, pheochromocytoma, and hyperparathyroidism.

A, B. MEN type IIb is associated with medullary thyroid carcinoma, pheochromocytoma, mucosal neuromas (neurofibromas), and a marfanoid body habitus.

C, D. Pancreatic tumors, such as insulinomas and pituitary tumors, are seen in association with MEN type I.

57. **A.** Medullary thyroid cancer (MTC) originates in the parafollicular cells, also known as the "C" cells of the thyroid gland. These cells are responsible for the production and secretion of calcitonin. Patients with pheochromocytomas and hypercalcemia should have a serum calcitonin level drawn to screen for MTC. An elevated level of calcitonin is seen in MTC.

B. Obtaining TSH levels is a step in evaluating functional thyroid disease, such as hyperthyroidism, but not in the case of thyroid cancers.

C. Serum calcium levels play no role in screening for MTC.

D. Ultrasound is useful in determining the character of the thyroid nodule, but it is not a screening tool for MTC.

E. FNA is used primarily as a safe, cost-effective diagnostic tool in the evaluation of thyroid nodules, when they are found. However, it is not useful for screening for MTC.

58. **C.** The RET gene has been implicated in the transmission of MEN type II syndromes.

A, B, D, E. MEN type II syndrome is not associated with these genes.

59. **C.** The parathyroid glands are derived embryologically from the third and fourth pharyngeal pouches. The inferior parathyroid glands arise from the dorsal portion of the third pouch and migrate inferiorly into the neck along with the thymus.

A. The first pharyngeal pouch will become the eustachian tube and middle ear.

B. The second pharyngeal pouch contributes to the development of the palatine tonsils.

D. The superior glands arise from the fourth pharyngeal pouch, and their migration is limited.

E. The fifth pharyngeal pouch is a rudimentary structure that becomes part of the fourth pouch.

60. **B.** Hepatic adenomas are benign lesions of the liver, most often found in women in their thirties and forties. Oral contraceptives are a risk factor for developing a hepatic adenoma. The lesions are usually solitary but can occur in multiples; they most often arise in the right lobe of the liver. Such lesions are often found incidentally on CT scan. Patients may present with abdominal pain and a palpable mass. The diagnosis can be made radiographically. A large adenoma of the right hepatic lobe is seen on the CT (see Figure 60; note arrow).

A. A hepatoma is a malignant tumor of the liver. It would be very uncommon in a young female with no history of cirrhosis of the liver.

C. Focal nodular hyperplasia is a benign liver tumor often seen in young women. It is associated with tissue ischemia and regeneration. Such a tumor appears as a central stellate scar on CT scan.

D. A hemangioendothelioma is a rare, benign lesion that usually appears in the first 2 years of life.

E. A hemangioma is the most frequently seen benign liver tumor. Most are small and asymptomatic. When they become larger, however, they can cause significant pain. Delayed-phase CT scan reveals pooling of contrast in the lesion, thus distinguishing it from other benign tumors.

61. **B.** Hepatic adenomas larger than 5 cm should be resected because one-third of patients present with bleeding or rupture of the adenoma.

A. Hepatic adenomas have a 10% risk of malignant degeneration.

C. A number of smaller adenomas may regress with cessation of the inciting agent—in this case, oral estrogens. Such cases may be followed rather than proceeding directly to surgery.

D. Acetaminophen is not a cause of hepatic adenomas, but can be related to liver damage as a result of overdosage.

E. Hepatic adenomas are not malignant and do not metastasize.

62. **B.** Superficial spreading is the most common type of melanoma, accounting for approximately 70% of melanomas. This lesion typically grows radially for months to years, having little surface elevation, but may eventually enter a vertical growth phase in which it develops a nodular component.

A. Lentigo maligna are cutaneous melanomas that are usually confined to chronically sun-damaged sites, such as the hands and neck. They are usually found in older adults and account for less than 10% of all melanomas.

C. Acral lentiginous are cutaneous melanomas that are usually found on the palms, soles of the feet, nail beds, and mucous membranes. They account for less than 10% of all melanomas.

D. Nodular melanomas do not grow radially, and usually present as deep, invasive lesions. They are dark brown-black or blue-black in color. They account for 15% to 30% of all melanomas.

E. Ocular melanomas are rare and often are not diagnosed until they become quite large. The most common site for them to develop is along the uveal tract. They account for 2% to 5% of all melanomas.

63. **C.** An insulinoma is a functional islet cell tumor that presents with symptoms of hypoglycemia (such as those described in this patient), often brought on by fasting or exercise. Other symptoms include palpitations, diaphoresis, tremulousness, irritability, weakness, vision changes, and neurologic changes. Carcinoid, gastrinoma, glucagonoma, somatostatinoma, and insulinoma are all forms of amine precursor uptake and decarboxylation (APUD) cell tumors.

A. Carcinoid tumor presentation symptoms can include diarrhea and flushing.

B. Gastrinoma tumor presentation symptoms can include abdominal pain and symptoms of acid hypersecretion.

D. Glucagonoma tumor presentation symptoms can include dermatitis, glucose intolerance or diabetes, and weight loss.

E. Somatostatinoma tumor presentation symptoms can include diabetes mellitus, gallbladder disease, diarrhea, and steatorrhea.

64. **D.** An insulinoma is diagnosed using a 72-hour fast followed by measurement of glucose, insulin, and C-peptide levels. An insulin/glucose ratio greater than 0.30 or an insulin level greater than 6 μU during a fast is diagnostic for an insulinoma.

A, B. CT scan and ultrasound of the abdomen are useful imaging tests, but because of the small size of insulinomas, they are successful only 50% of the time in localizing the lesion. Angiography with subtraction techniques or intraoperative ultrasound are the two most accurate tests.

C. A euglycemic C-peptide suppression test may be useful, but it is rarely used.

E. Diazoxide (Hyperstat) is used to inhibit insulin release and to decrease peripheral glucose utilization. Secondary to its multiple side effects, it is used for a short period to help briefly control symptoms and is inappropriate until the diagnosis of insulinoma has been made.

65. **B.** Whipple's triad consists of hypoglycemic symptoms with fasting, blood glucose less than 50 mg/dL, and relief of symptoms with administration of glucose. It is associated with an insulinoma diagnosis.

A. Beck's triad (shock, distant heart sounds, and distended neck veins) is associated with pericardial tamponade.

C. Charcot's triad (jaundice, fever, and upper quadrant pain) is associated with cholangitis.

D. Virchow's triad (abnormal vessel wall, circulating blood abnormalities, and stasis) is associated with venous thrombosis.

E. There is no such thing as Ostlund's triad.

66. **C.** A neuroblastoma is the most common childhood solid, malignant tumor. The majority of patients present with an asymptomatic abdominal mass. These tumors most often arise in the adrenal gland, originating from neural crest cells of the adrenal medulla or sympathetic chain.

A. The neck is the least common location for a neuroblastoma.

B. The mediastinum is the second most common location for a neuroblastoma.

D. Neuroblastomas are not found in the spleen.

E. The third most common location for a neuroblastoma is in the pelvis.

67. **A.** The stage of the tumor is determined by the size, such as a tumor crossing the midline, nodal status, and distant metastases. Patients with a Stage I neuroblastoma have a 100% survival rate with therapy. Radiotherapy is used only when incomplete excision has been performed. Preoperative chemoradiation is used when the tumor appears unresectable on imaging studies. Staging and survival rates are listed in Table 67.

B, C, D, E. These factors are unrelated to staging the tumor.

TABLE 67 Neuroblastoma Staging

Stage	Survival Rate with Therapy
I: Confined to the origin	100%
IIa: Completely excised unilateral tumor, (–) nodes	80%
IIb: Completely excised unilateral tumor, (+) nodes	70%
III: Tumor across midline or contralateral (+) nodes	40%
IV: Distant metastasis	15%

68. **B.** Amplification of the n-myc gene correlates with poor outcomes in neuroblastomas.

A. The k-ras gene is associated with colorectal, lung, and prostate cancer.

C. The c-abl gene is associated with the Philadelphia chromosome in CML.

D. The protein HER-2/neu is overexpressed in approximately 20% to 30% of breast cancers.

E. The c-myc gene is associated with Burkitt's lymphoma.

69. **C.** This patient presents with a partial small bowel obstruction (SBO). In the setting of previous abdominal surgery, the most likely cause of the obstruction is an adhesive band. The leading cause of SBO in developed countries is postoperative adhesions, which account for approximately 50% to 70% of all cases. Surgeries most commonly related to SBO are appendectomy, upper gastrointestinal, colorectal, and gynecologic procedures. Small bowel obstructions can be partial or complete.

A. Primary small bowel tumors are an extremely rare cause of partial bowel obstruction. Neoplasms account for approximately 10% of cases.

B. Metastatic ovarian cancer to the bowel is a cause of partial bowel obstruction. Given that adhesive bands are the cause of 50% to 70% of all SBOs in patients with previous abdominal surgery, metastatic cancer is less likely in this case.

D. Hernias are the second most common cause of partial obstructions, accounting for approximately 25% of all cases. They are the most common cause in patients who have not undergone prior abdominal surgery.

E. An ileus is a mechanical or functional intestinal obstruction resulting in dysfunctional motility of the bowel. It is most commonly seen immediately following abdominal surgery, in patients with metabolic abnormalities, or with infectious processes. The x-ray findings in this case are not consistent with an ileus.

70. **D.** Initial nonoperative management of a partial SBO includes strict bowel rest, nasogastric tube (NGT) decompression, IV fluids, and placement of a Foley catheter to monitor urine output closely.

A. Total parenteral nutrition is not part of the initial management of SBO.

B. NGT placement is indicated in all except mild cases of SBO. It will decompress the stomach, eliminate vomiting, minimize discomfort of reflux of intestinal contents, and assist in monitoring intestinal output.

C. Antibiotics do not have a role in the initial management of SBO. They will, however, have a role if the patient requires surgery.

E. Medical management or nonoperative management for SBO is prudent and appropriate. Most episodes of obstructions from adhesions resolve without surgical intervention.

71. **E.** The four cardinal signs indicating the need for prompt operative intervention are persistent focal tenderness, fever, leukocytosis, and tachycardia. Given this patient's current findings, she should go directly to the operating room for exploratory laparotomy.

A, B, C, D. These are all inappropriate choices in this scenario because this patient has failed conservative management of a bowel obstruction and has now deteriorated as indicated by the leukocytosis, tachycardia, fever, and persistent focal tenderness.

72. **D.** Ninety percent of bladder cancers are transitional cell tumors, with the remainder being either squamous cell or adenocarcinoma. Men are more prone to developing bladder cancer than are women. The risk of developing bladder cancer is increased by smoking and exposure to β-naphthylamine and/or paraminodiphenyl. Treatment of T0 and T1 tumors includes transurethral resection of the bladder tumor with or without chemotherapy.

A. The use of postoperative radiation therapy is controversial; it is considered only in T2 and T3 stage disease.

B. Chemotherapy alone is not sufficient; resection of the tumor is required.

C. Chemotherapy and radiation therapy alone are not sufficient; resection of the tumor is required.

E. Radical cystectomy is indicated in stage T2 and T3 tumors.

73. **B.** Patients with kidney stone disease usually present with acute onset of pain in the flank that radiates to the groin. The patient is often unable to find a comfortable position, and vomiting is common. Dysuria, frequency, and hematuria may be present. Evaluation of the urine will reveal hematuria unless the affected ureter is totally obstructed. An abdominal x-ray may be helpful because 90% of stones are radio-opaque. Most commonly, a CT scan without contrast is used to evaluate for stones. Pain is usually severe. Although this patient is a known narcotic abuser, narcotic pain medication should not be withheld with objective proof that the patient is actually suffering from nephrolithiasis. Figure 73B shows the CT scan typically ordered to rule out kidney stones; note the arrow, which points to a nephrolith.

A. An emergent ureteroscopy may be needed if the patient is unable to pass the stones due to their size. The initial therapy, however, is IV fluid hydration and pain control.

C. There is no indication at this time for an exploratory laparotomy.

D. NSAIDs are a reasonable choice, but the pain relief they offer would most likely be insufficient.

E. This patient has clinical and radiographic signs of kidney stone disease and should be treated appropriately, regardless of the history of narcotic abuse.

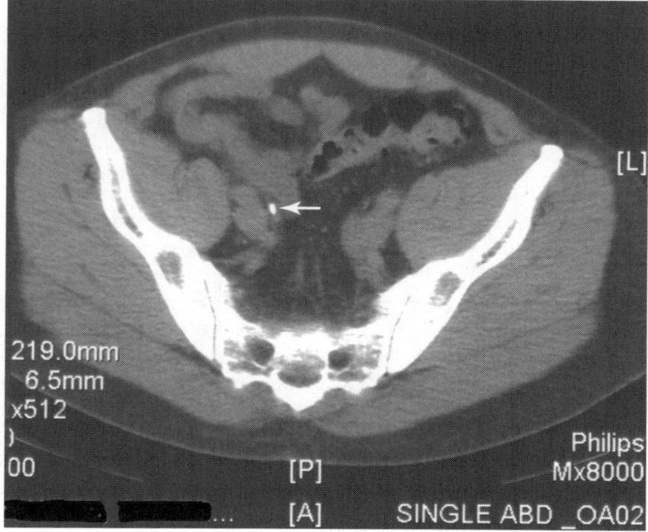

Figure 73B • Image courtesy of the University of Utah School of Medicine, Salt Lake City, Utah.

74. **B.** Kidney stones are most commonly calcium phosphate and calcium oxalate (80%), struvite (15%), uric acid (5%), and cystine (1%). Calcium and struvite stones are more common in women. Uric acid stones are twice as common in men, and cystine stones occur in both men and women with the same frequency. Absorptive hyperoxaluria occurs in approximately 10% of people who have undergone surgical removal of a portion of the bowel. It causes unabsorbed fatty acids to combine with calcium. This results in excess oxalate absorption by the gut, resulting in formation of calcium oxalate stones.

A. Uric acid stones are found in approximately 5% of cases. These radiolucent stones are associated with gout, Lesch-Nyhan syndrome, and a low urine pH.

C. Cystine stones are rare, being found in fewer than 1% of cases. Affected individuals have a genetic predisposition for developing such stones.

D. Struvite stones are composed of magnesium, ammonia, and phosphate. They occur in approximately 15% of cases and are associated with UTIs with urea-splitting bacteria, such as *Proteus* and *Pseudomonas.* Infection with these organisms may cause staghorn calculi that fill the entire renal pelvis.

E. Cysteine is not a component of kidney stones.

75. **B.** Gastric adenocarcinoma encompasses 90% to 95% of all gastric tumors. It is the eighth most common cause of cancer mortality in the United States. This type of cancer is seen more frequently in males than in females (2:1 ratio), and 70% of patients are more than 50 years old. The incidence of gastric cancer is highest in Asia, with the incidence in Japan being 80 times higher than the incidence in the United States. Risk factors include diet (smoked foods), exposure to nitrosamine compounds, low consumption of fruits and vegetables, occupational exposures (heavy metals, rubber, and asbestos), cigarette smoking, alcohol use, and low socioeconomic status.

A, C. Chewing tobacco and high-fat diets are not associated with an increased risk for developing gastric cancer.

D. While the Japanese do have a much higher incidence, it is believed to be due to their diet and is not a genetic-related risk.

E. See the explanation for B.

76. **C.** Tumors can be located anywhere in the stomach, although there is a general pattern to their distribution. Thirty percent are located in the pyloric canal or antrum, 20% to 30% in the body, 37% in the cardia, and 12% in the entire stomach (Linitis plastica). Many remember the distribution as approximately one-third in the antrum, one-third in the body, and one-third in the cardia. The corpus is another name for the body of the stomach.

A, B, D, E. These distribution patterns are incorrect. See the explanation for C.

77. **C.** Continuous bleeding from the rectum with or without hemodynamic instability is known as an acute lower GI hemorrhage. This patient appears stable, as evidenced by the stable vital signs and unchanged hematocrit. Nevertheless, the patient should be closely observed. A nasogastric tube should be placed to rule out the possibility of rapid upper GI bleeding. Once this diagnosis is ruled out, the patient should have a colonoscopy to help determine the cause of lower GI bleeding. According to the results of clinical trials, colonoscopy is successful in localizing the bleeding sites 50% to 90% of the time. Therapy consisting of cauterization can also be employed if the site of active bleeding is identified.

A. Diagnostic laparoscopy would not be helpful in this situation, as the source of the bleeding usually cannot be identified by simply looking into the abdomen with a laparoscope. A localizing study, such as a colonoscopy, should be performed first.

B. A CT scan would not be helpful in diagnosing the source of ongoing bleeding within the colon.

D. Angiography may be used to localize the bleeding vessel and treat it by embolization. Identification in this manner typically requires a fairly rapid rate of bleeding to localize the source of bleeding. This procedure is more invasive than colonoscopy and would not be the first choice. It is an option, however, if the bleeding cannot be controlled at the time of colonoscopy.

E. Exploratory laparotomy may be required in an unstable patient after unsuccessful endoscopy. If the source of bleeding is not localized, a total colectomy may be the only option.

78. **E.** There are multiple causes of lower GI bleeding, with the most common etiology in the United States being diverticulosis. Approximately 80% to 90% of lower GI bleeds stop spontaneously, with a 25% rate of rebleeding. It is imperative to attempt to localize and treat the underlying disorder to prevent any future bleeding.

A. Inflammatory bowel disease is the fourth most common cause of lower GI bleeding.

B. Neoplasms are the fifth most common cause of lower GI bleeding.

C. Meckel's diverticulum is the sixth most common cause of lower GI bleeding.

D. Vascular ectasia is the second most common cause of lower GI bleeding.

79. **E.** The splenic vein empties into the portal vein directly.

A. The inferior mesenteric vein empties into the splenic vein.

B. The superior mesenteric vein empties into the portal vein.

C. Blood returns to the vena cava after going through the liver and out the hepatic veins to the vena cava.

D. The azygous vein empties into the superior vena cava in the chest.

80. **A.** Immunologic function of the spleen is needed to prevent overwhelming infections from encapsulated bacteria such as *Streptococcus pneumoniae, Haemophilus influenzae,* and *Meningococcus*. When considering splenectomy, patients should receive vaccinations protecting against all of these organisms. This measure helps to prevent the condition known as overwhelming post-splenectomy infection (OPSI), which can be fatal. Children are more susceptible to this complication and are often kept on prophylactic antibiotics.

B. A preoperative CT scan is not needed, either to evaluate splenic size, which is usually near normal in AHA, or to look for other problems.

C. Platelet count and function are not affected in AHA, and transfusion of platelets should not be necessary.

D. Today, most normal-sized spleens would be removed laparoscopically. There is no advantage to open surgery in the evaluation for accessory spleens.

E. Unless pancreatic injury or other unusual complications occurs, the routine use of left upper quadrant (LUQ) drains is not needed.

81. **A.** A patient who is post-splenectomy and who presents with an increased number of platelets (greater than 1,000,000) should be started on aspirin to prevent spontaneous clotting. Aspirin does not destroy platelets, but rather makes them dysfunctional and thus decreases the risk of thrombus formation.

B, C, D. Systemic anticoagulation is not necessary, nor are preventive doses of Coumadin or Lovenox, as long as the patient can continue to take aspirin.

E. The increased risk of spontaneous thrombus formation requires treatment.

82. **D.** A solitary rectal ulcer is an uncommon cause of acute rectal pain and is thought to be due to excessive straining during which the anterior rectal mucosa is forced into the anal canal, causing congestion, edema, and ulceration.

A. A perirectal abscess typically causes severe anal pain, worsened by defecation. Diagnosis is made by rectal exam and palpation of an indurated perirectal mass.

B. Rectal neoplasms tend to be occult in terms of symptoms; they do not cause sudden acute pain.

C. An anal fissure occurs after forceful dilatation of the anal canal. It usually occurs after constipation with forceful defecation. An anal fissure most frequently occurs in the posterior midline, leading to increasing pain with defecation and reluctance to have further bowel movements. This results in further constipation, which in turn worsens the problem. The diagnosis is made by simply separating the buttocks, revealing a tear in the anoderm of the posterior midline.

E. Anal condylomata are caused by infection with human papillomavirus (HPV) types 6 and 11. Affected individuals complain of a perianal growth that appears as a cauliflower-like lesion on physical exam. Minimal disease may be treated in the office with bichloracetic acid or podophyllum; larger lesions may require surgical excision.

83. **A.** The goals of treatment for a solitary rectal ulcer (SRU) include patient reassurance that the lesion is benign and cessation or minimization of symptoms, which can be achieved with conservative therapy consisting of dietary fiber, stool softeners, bowel retraining, and bulking agents.

B. Narcotic pain medication is often needed, and it should be used in conjunction with stool softeners. Narcotics should be used conservatively, as they may increase the patient's constipation.

C. Surgical treatment is an option, and it is typically indicated for those patients who fail conservative management.

D. An exam under anesthesia is not required as part of intitial therapy.

E. Nitroglycerin topical ointment has been reported to be an effective treatment for anal fissures but not for SRU. Its use is limited because of the high incidence of side effects, which include headaches and tachyphylaxis.

84. **A.** For patients who fail dietary measures, a trial of sucralfate enemas is the next therapeutic step. A rectopexy or other surgical procedure should be reserved for failures of all other measures.

B. Abdominoperineal resection is used to treat rectal tumors less than 5 cm from the anal verge.

C. Lateral internal anal sphincterotomy is the procedure of choice after failure of medical management for anal fissures, not SRU. In this procedure the internal anal sphincter is divided, relieving the spasm that causes pain and limits healing. Fecal continence is maintained by the external anal sphincter. This procedure has a success rate exceeding 90%.

D. A low anterior resection is used to treat rectal cancer that is more than 5 cm from the anal verge.

E. While a diverting colostomy might allow the SRU to heal, it is a morbid operation and requires a second operation.

85. **B.** Prostate cancer is the most common neoplasm, after skin cancer, in men and the second most common cause of cancer-related death. Prostate cancer occurs more commonly in African American men and in men older than age 50. Ninety-five percent of prostate tumors involve adenocarcinoma, and they occur primarily in the peripheral zone. A transrectal ultrasound is used to evaluate tumor volume and aid the acquisition of biopsies.

A. A cystoscopy with washings is not required except in cases of large lesions with suspected bladder involvement.

C. A pelvic CT scan will most likely eventually be required to assist in the staging of this disease, but it would not be the initial step in this patient's management.

D. Because the patient's history and physical exam are very concerning for prostate cancer, further diagnostic evaluation is warranted, not observation.

E. A pelvic MRI has no role in the initial work-up of prostate cancer.

86. **C.** Patients with nonpalpable tumors and more than 5% prostate involvement (stage A2), or with localized nodules of 1 to 1.5 cm in diameter in one lobe (stage B1), or with a tumor greater than 1.5 cm in diameter in one or more lobes (stage B2) are candidates for total prostatectomy.

A. Observation is usually reserved for stage A1 disease, which includes nonpalpable tumors with an incidental finding of low-grade cancer seen in less than 5% of the prostate.

B. Radiation therapy is used in stage C disease, which includes periprostatic extension of tumor.

D. Hormonal therapy alone should be used in men with stage D cancer, which consists of distant metastases.

E. Pelvic MRI has no role in the initial work-up for, or treatment of, prostate cancer.

87. **D.** Any patient with a history of prostate cancer and elevated alkaline phosphatase should be evaluated for metastatic disease to the bones. Prostate metastases cause osteoblastic lesions. Treatment is usually palliative and consists of hormonal therapy and irradiation of symptomatic lesions.

A. Sarcoidosis is a disease of unknown etiology characterized by noncaseating granulomas in multiple tissues. Hypercalcemia results from excessive secretion of $1{,}25(OH)_2D_3$ and occurs in 20% of patients.

B. Metastatic prostate cancer results in hypercalcemia due to osteoblastic—not osteoclastic—bone metastases.

C. Cholestasis refers to delay or obstruction of bile secretion. It does not cause elevated calcium levels.

E. Vitamin D deficiency results in hypocalcemia. Dietary rickets is uncommon today in the United States, especially since vitamin D has been added to milk products.

88. **E.** The most common—albeit rare—primary malignant bone tumor is osteogenic sarcoma. Males between 10 and 20 years of age are most often affected. The lesion occurs on the metaphysis of the distal femur or proximal tibia. The presenting symptoms are usually pain, tenderness, and swelling near a joint. Limitation of motion may also be present. Serum alkaline phosphatase is usually elevated, and plain films reveal a destructive lesion in the metaphysis area of long bones with periosteal elevation known as Codman's triangle.

A. An osteoclastoma is a benign tumor that contains highly vascular cellular stroma and occurs on the ends of long bones. Radiographically they appear as clear cystic tumors. Treatment is via surgical excision, and the local recurrence rate is as high as 50%.

B. Ewing's sarcoma is a small, round, blue cell malignancy that occurs at the diaphysis of long bones. Affected individuals are usually younger than 20 years of age. The radiographic characteristic of "onion-skinning" is caused by the tumor extending from the medulla with new bone formation parallel to the shaft. This tumor is extremely malignant, with early metastases being observed.

C. Chondrosarcomas arise from chondroblasts and usually occur in older age groups. They are found most commonly in the pelvis, ribs, sternum, or femur. Plain films demonstrate destruction of the involved bone with an expanding soft tissue mass containing irregular calcifications.

D. Unicameral bone cysts are common benign bone cysts of uncertain etiology, which most often arise during childhood. The lesions are often asymptomatic and discovered incidentally, although some may present as pathologic fractures. The most frequent site for their development is the proximal humeral metaphysis. Radiographically one observes a well-defined metaphyseal lucency that may expand the bone. Small cysts may be treated with steroid injections; larger cysts may require surgical curettage and bone grafting.

89. **E.** Patients born with familial retinoblastoma inherit a defective copy of the retinoblastoma (RB) tumor suppressor gene located on chromosome 13q14. Mutation of the normal RB gene early in development leads to the emergence of retinoblastoma at an early age. Treatment is surgical excision. These children are at an increased risk for developing an osteogenic sarcoma and other soft tissue sarcomas.

A. Neurofibromatosis, also known as Von Recklinghausen's disease, is associated with multiple neurofibromas of the skin. Affected individuals also have café au lait spots. This disease is associated with pheochromocytomas and osteitis fibrosa cystica. There is no association with osteosarcoma.

B, C, D. Premature birth, history of loose, bloody stools, and prior broken bones are all nonspecific findings.

90. **A.** The natural history of an osteogenic sarcoma is relentless growth, early metastasis to the lungs, and death if not appropriately and aggressively treated. Current therapy combines limb salvage surgery with preoperative and postoperative chemotherapy consisting of multiple cytotoxic drugs. The 5-year survival rate is greater than 70% with this therapy.

B. At one point, radiation with delayed amputation was the standard treatment for osteosarcoma, with a 5-year survival rate of less than 20%.

C. Osteosarcomas are often radiation resistant. For that reason, radiation therapy is now limited to large, unresectable tumors.

D, E. Limb-sparing surgery is the current standard of care in the treatment of this tumor.

91. **D.** While this patient initially presented with what might appear to be acute cholecystitis, this condition has progressed to an acute abdomen. The patient needs to be emergently taken to the operating room for exploratory abdominal surgery.

A, C. Regardless of any new radiographic study finding, based on the clinical signs of an acute abdomen, the patient needs to be emergently taken to the operating room.

B. Increasing pain medication will make the patient comfortable, but it will not solve the underlying problem. If the patient has been given too much medication, it may affect the ability to truly evaluate her clinical abdominal exam.

E. Fluid boluses may be required as a result of the global inflammatory response seen with an acute abdomen, in which the fluid requirements increase. The patient should be closely followed, with frequent monitoring of her vital signs and urine output.

92. **C.** This case involves a type III ulcer, which is located in the prepyloric region of the stomach.

A. A type I ulcer is located along the lesser curvature of the stomach.

B. A type II ulcer is a combination of an ulcer in the body of the stomach and a duodenal ulcer.

D. A type IV ulcer is an ulcer at the gastroesophageal junction.

E. There is no type V ulcer category.

93. **D.** Because type III ulcers are less likely to be associated with hyperacidity and can carry a risk of being malignant, removal of the ulcer via a distal gastrectomy without vagotomy is the best choice.

A. A vagotomy and pyloroplasty is a procedure used for management of peptic ulcer disease. This approach would not remove the ulcer for pathologic evaluation.

B. While a total gastrectomy would obviously remove the ulcer, this procedure involves significant morbidity not justified in this scenario.

C. A highly selective vagotomy is a procedure used to lower acidity in peptic ulcer disease. It would not be indicated in treatment of type III ulcers and would not allow pathologic evaluation of the ulcer.

E. Vagotomy and gastrojejunostomy is a procedure that was used and then discarded as an acid-reducing strategy. It would not be appropriate in this case and would not remove the ulcer for pathologic examination.

F. Proximal gastric resection would not remove the ulcer and is not a standard gastric procedure. Therefore it is inappropriate in this case.

94. **C.** Afferent loop syndrome presents with postprandial distention, nausea, and RUQ pain, all of which are relieved by emesis, typically bilious in nature. The acute form may be due to edema at the gastrojejunostomy, obstructing the afferent loop. If symptoms persist, conversion to a Roux-en-Y gastrojejunostomy may be required.

A. Recurrent ulcers are more common with duodenal ulcers and occur at the anastomotic site. They usually present with pain and postprandial vomiting.

B. Postprandial dumping syndrome is the most common complication of gastrectomy. Symptoms include pain, vomiting, diarrhea, palpitations, and flushing usually within 30 minutes of a meal.

D. Postvagotomy diarrhea occurs episodically and may be associated with nausea and vomiting. Typical treatment consists of dietary adjustments and antidiarrheals.

E. Bile reflux gastritis presents with epigastric pain associated with nausea and vomiting. Initial therapy consists of H_2 blockers.

95. **B.** Early postprandial dumping syndrome is the most common postgastrectomy complication. Rapid emptying of hyperosmolar chyme causes intravascular fluid shifts, resulting in symptoms that include pain, vomiting, diarrhea, palpitations, and flushing usually within 30 minutes of a meal. Frequent consumption of high-protein, low-carbohydrate meals is recommended to decrease the incidence and severity of this syndrome.

A. Recurrent ulcers are more common with duodenal ulcers and occur at the anastomotic site. They usually present with pain and postprandial vomiting.

C. Afferent loop syndrome presents with postprandial distention, nausea, and RUQ pain, which are relieved by emesis, typically bilious in nature.

D. Late postprandial dumping syndrome is also known as reactive hypoglycemia. Ingestion of large amounts of carbohydrates stimulates insulin release, causing hypoglycemia several hours after eating.

E. Bile reflux gastritis presents with epigastric pain associated with nausea and vomiting. Initial therapy consists of H_2 blockers.

96. **D.** This patient's history and physical exam are concerning for a possible choledochal cyst. A choledochal cyst is a congenital malformation of the bile ducts that results in cystic dilations. Five types of choledochal cysts exist:

- I: Dilation of the common bile duct
- II: Diverticulum of the common bile duct
- III: Choledochocele
- IV: Multiple intrahepatic and extrahepatic choledochocysts
- V: Single or multiple intrahepatic cysts (Caroli disease)

Patients present with a triad of symptoms: recurrent abdominal pain, mild episodic jaundice, and a right upper quadrant mass. Choledochal cysts are frequently seen in older children. Excision of the cyst is the treatment of choice.

A. Acute cholecystitis is an unlikely choice, based on the child's age, history, and physical exam.

B. Acute cholangitis in a child without a fever is unlikely.

C. A mass in the head of the pancreas would be an unlikely choice, for the same reason of age, as well as the episodic jaundice. A mass of the pancreas would be more likely to present with persistent jaundice.

E. Choledocholithiasis is a possibility, but the history is not consistent with biliary colic and this condition would be less likely at this age. Obtaining an ultrasound of the right upper quadrant would be the study of choice, and would help eliminate this possibility.

97. **A.** The initial study of choice is a right upper quadrant ultrasound. Diagnosis can often be made from an ultrasound alone. Other studies, such as an abdominal CT scan, hepatobiliary scintigraphy, ERCP, or cholangiography, may be obtained later as needed to formulate a treatment plan.

B. An abdominal CT scan would not be considered the initial diagnostic study in this case.

C. Hepatobiliary scintigraphy is useful in detecting associated intrahepatic cystic disease or obstruction, but in this scenario it is not the initial study of choice.

D. An ERCP would be useful later to define the location of the cyst and to aid in placement of a stent if necessary.

E. Cholangiography is used to define the anatomy and location of the cyst. It would be performed secondary to an initial ultrasound of the right upper quadrant.

98. **A.** The most common primary malignant tumor of the liver is hepatocellular carcinoma (HCC). It is also one of the most common solid cancers in the world, with an annual incidence estimated at 1 million new patients per year. Patients with cirrhosis, hepatitis B, history of alcohol abuse, hemochromatosis, schistosomiasis, aflatoxin, and α-1-antitrypsin disease all have an increased risk of developing HCC. Patients typically present with dull RUQ pain, weight loss, hepatomegaly, and an abdominal mass. Treatment consists of surgical resection if possible. Unfortunately, only 5% to 15% of newly diagnosed patients with HCC undergo a potentially curative resection. Figure 98 shows an obvious tumor in the right lobe of the liver.

B. While cholangiocarcinoma is included in the differential diagnosis, it accounts for only 7% of all primary hepatic tumors. Cholangiocarcinoma is associated with chronic cholestasis, congenital cystic disease of the liver, and infection with the liver fluke, *Clonorchis sinensis.* Given this patient's history of cirrhosis and alcohol abuse, HCC is a more likely diagnosis.

C. A hepatoblastoma is a tumor seen in infants and children.

D. A hemangioma is a benign liver tumor, which rarely causes symptoms such as presented in this case.

E. An adenoma is a benign lesion that occurs primarily in young females taking oral contraceptives.

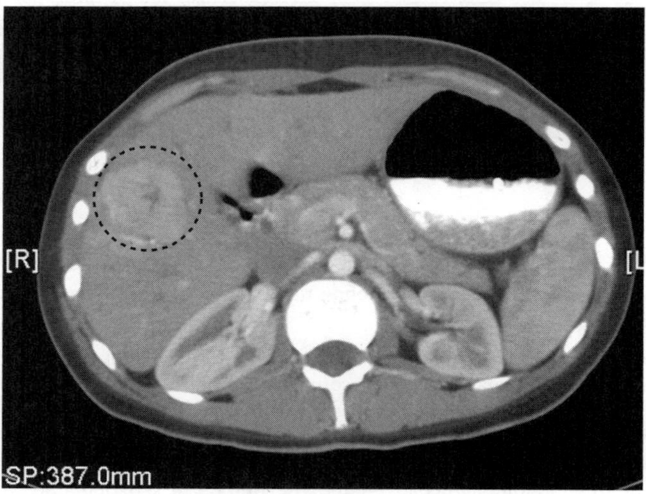

Figure 98 • Image courtesy of the University of Utah School of Medicine, Salt Lake City, Utah.

99. **B.** Alpha fetoprotein (AFP) is associated with hepatocellular carcinoma. More than 70% of patients with an HCC larger than 3 cm will have an elevated AFP level.

A. β-hCG is associated with intrauterine pregnancy, as well as testicular and trophoblastic tumors.

C. CA 19-9 is associated with pancreatic cancer; it may also be elevated in colorectal and gastric cancers.

D. CEA is associated with colorectal cancer; it may also be elevated in HCC, pancreatic, breast, and testicular cancers.

E. CA 125 is associated with ovarian tumors.

100. **E.** The most common site of distant metastasis for a hepatocellular carcinoma is to the lungs. Local invasion into the diaphragm is also common.

A, B, C, D. The brain, spleen, small bowel, and pancreas are unlikely locations for metastasis of HCC.

Block

THREE

Questions

Setting 3: Inpatient Facilities

You have general admitting privileges to the hospital. You may see patients in the critical care unit, the pediatrics unit, the maternity unit, or recovery room. You may also be called to see patients in the psychiatric unit. A short-stay unit serves patients who are undergoing same-day operations or who are being held for observation. There are adjacent nursing home/extended-care facilities and a detoxification unit where you may see patients.

101. A 3-day-old male infant is transferred to the newborn intensive care unit from an outside facility with abdominal distention, bilious emesis, and failure to pass meconium. You evaluate the infant and, after obtaining a contrast enema (Figure 101A), determine that he has meconium ileus. Which other condition is this child at risk for having?

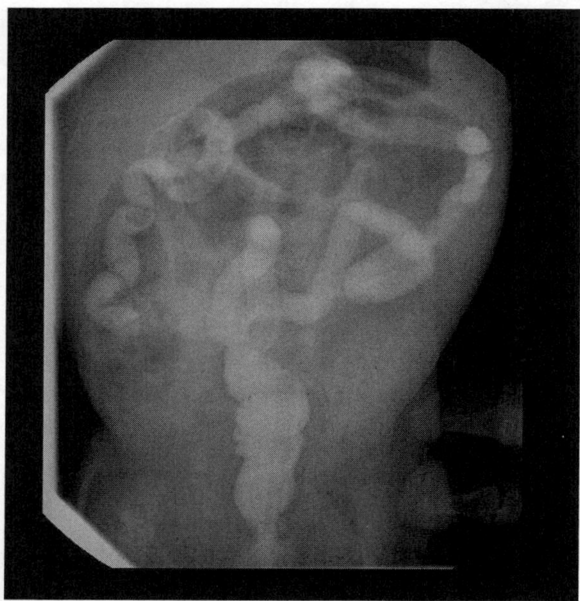

Figure 101A • Image courtesy of the University of Utah School of Medicine, Salt Lake City, Utah.

A. Budd-Chiari syndrome
B. Down syndrome
C. von Hippel-Lindau syndrome
D. Eaton-Lambert syndrome
E. Cystic fibrosis

102. You are called to the newborn intensive care unit to evaluate a 36-hour-old infant whose abdomen has become distended, associated with bilious emesis. After performing your history and physical exam, you obtain an abdominal x-ray (Figure 102A). What is the most likely diagnosis in this case?

A. Midgut volvulus
B. Hypertrophic pyloric stenosis
C. Duodenal atresia
D. Intestinal malrotation
E. Hirschsprung's disease

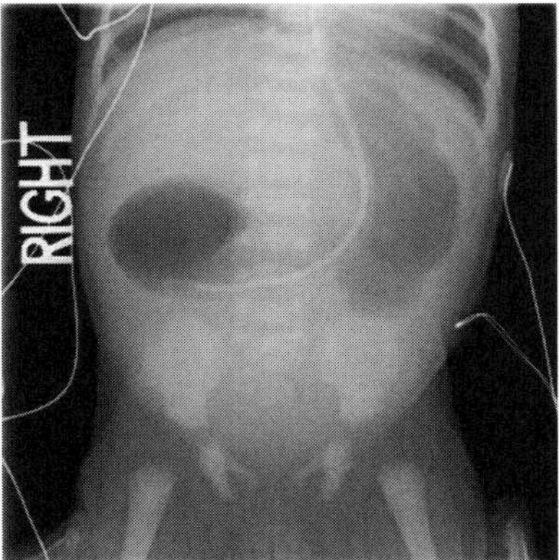

Figure 102A • Image courtesy of the University of Utah School of Medicine, Salt Lake City, Utah.

The next three questions (items 103–105) correspond to the following vignette.

A 50-year-old female patient scheduled to be discharged from the hospital the next day is suffering from an unrelated 2-week history of extreme pain upon defecation. The patient denies any associated abdominal pain, nausea, vomiting, fever, or chills. She reports a long history of constipation, which has been severe lately. She has also noticed slight spotting of blood on tissue paper, but denies any anal drainage, bright red blood per rectum, or melena.

103. On examination, what is the most likely physical finding in this patient?

- **A.** Disruption of anoderm in the posterior midline.
- **B.** Protrusion of an internal hemorrhoid
- **C.** Fistula in ano
- **D.** Perirectal abscess
- **E.** Anal condyloma

104. What is the best initial therapy for this patient?

- **A.** Surgical treatment
- **B.** 0.2% nitroglycerin topical ointment
- **C.** Stool softeners, bulking agents, and sitz baths
- **D.** Botulinum toxin
- **E.** No treatment is necessary

105. The patient returns to your outpatient office with the same complaints and physical findings 6 weeks after completing initial management. What is the next best step in the management of this patient's problem?

- **A.** Diverting colostomy
- **B.** Lateral internal anal sphincterotomy
- **C.** Low anterior resection
- **D.** Incision and drainage
- **E.** Hemorrhoidectomy

End of set

106. You are called to evaluate a 33-year-old female on the cardiology service who recently delivered a healthy baby girl. During the course of her pregnancy, the patient developed dilated cardiomyopathy that progressed to complete heart failure. The patient has remained in the cardiac intensive care unit on multiple inotropes, which the cardiologists have been unable to wean. The patient recently had a balloon pump placed. The transplant cardiology service is likewise seeing this young woman to evaluate for a heart transplant. What is the next best option you could offer this patient prior to receiving a transplant?

- **A.** Aortic valve replacement
- **B.** Placement of a biventricular assist device
- **C.** Coronary artery bypass grafting
- **D.** Extracorporeal membrane oxygenation (ECMO)
- **E.** Vigorous diuresis and physical therapy

107. A 66-year-old male is undergoing coronary artery bypass grafting to the left anterior descending, circumflex, and right coronary arteries. Despite maximizing volume status and optimizing inotropic agents, the patient is unable to be weaned from the cardiopulmonary bypass machine, at which time an intra-aortic balloon pump is placed. Which of the following statements is true regarding intra-aortic balloon pumps?

- **A.** They decrease afterload by inflating during systole.
- **B.** They augment coronary artery flow during diastole.
- **C.** They assist in afterload reduction in aortic regurgitation.
- **D.** They increase mesenteric flow by inflating during systole.
- **E.** Immediate postoperative use is contraindicated secondary to bleeding risks.

The next three questions (items 108–110) correspond to the following vignette.

The orthopedic surgery service asks you to evaluate a 78-year-old female who underwent total hip replacement 8 days ago. The patient was initially tolerating her diet, but over the last 3 days she has become distended and has begun having nausea and vomiting. On exam, the patient's abdomen is distended and nontender.

108. Based on the abdominal film shown (Figure 108), what is the most likely diagnosis?

- **A.** Ogilvie syndrome
- **B.** Acute SBO
- **C.** Toxic megacolon
- **D.** *C. difficile* colitis
- **E.** Mesenteric ischemia

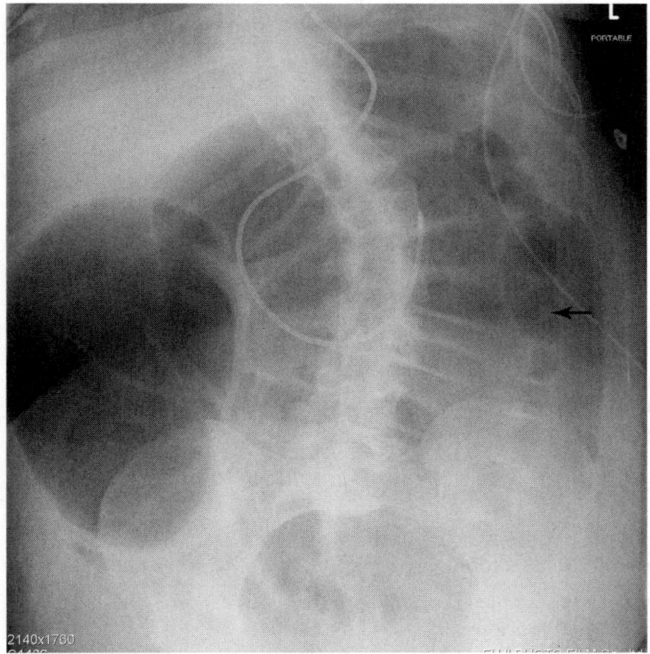

Figure 108 • Image courtesy of the University of Utah School of Medicine, Salt Lake City, Utah

109. What is the best initial approach to this patient's problem?

- **A.** Immediate exploratory laparotomy
- **B.** IV antibiotics and proton pump inhibitors
- **C.** Total parenteral nutrition
- **D.** Institution of nasojejunal feedings
- **E.** Neostigmine

110. Prior to treatment, the patient should have correction of serum electrolytes and which of the following procedures?

- **A.** Chest x-ray
- **B.** ECG
- **C.** Continuous pulse oximetry
- **D.** Continuous cardiac monitoring
- **E.** Baseline arterial blood gas

End of set

The next two questions (items 111 and 112) correspond to the following vignette.

You are called to see a 73-year-old male in the medical ICU for evaluation of a GI bleed. The medicine service intern reports that bright red blood was first noticed in the patient's stool this morning. Throughout the day, the patient has become progressively more tachycardic despite a 250 cc bolus of normal saline (NS). The patient has a history of colon cancer, which was resected via a left hemicolectomy 8 years ago. The vital signs are as follows: BP 110/72, HR 116, and RR 14. You examine the patient, and see that he has difficulty talking due to the CPAP mask he is wearing. The rectal exam is unremarkable except for gross blood. You place a central line in order to have large bore access for fluids.

111. What is the first step in this patient's management?

A. Barium enema
B. Placement of an NGT
C. Rigid proctoscopy
D. Colonoscopy
E. Urgent operative procedure

112. You choose to send the patient to angiography for embolization of the bleeding vessel. What is the main limiting factor of angiography?

A. Difficult to visualize if the bleed is in the proximal duodenum
B. Difficult to visualize if it is a small bowel bleed
C. Difficult to visualize if the bleed is less than 1 cc/min
D. Difficult to visualize if cauterization was attempted during colonoscopy
E. Difficult to localize recurrent tumor by angiography

End of set

---

113. During an elective repair of a right inguinal hernia in a 6-year-old male, an undescended testicle is encountered in the inguinal canal. In addition to a high ligation repair of the indirect hernia sac, an orchiopexy is performed. Which of the following statements is true regarding testicular tumors?

A. Germ cell tumors are the least common type of testicular cancer.
B. An elevated serum human chorionic gonadotropin (hCG) level is almost always found in association with seminoma.
C. Orchiopexy does not reduce the likelihood that this patient will develop testicular cancer.
D. A biopsy of suspected testicular cancer may be safely performed under local anesthesia via a scrotal incision.
E. Seminomas are insensitive to radiation therapy.

The next three questions (items 114–116) correspond to the following vignette.

An 81-year-old male undergoes an elective abdominal aortic aneurysm repair. The surgery is uncomplicated, and the patient is transported to the SICU in guarded condition. When the patient is examined on postoperative day 1, he is unable to move his legs. There is decreased sensation to both the posterior and anterior aspects of his legs, and rectal sphincter tone is absent.

114. What is the most appropriate next step in the work-up of this patient?

- **A.** Electromyography of the lower extremities
- **B.** Lumbar puncture
- **C.** MRI of the spinal cord
- **D.** CT scan of the head
- **E.** Lumbar myelogram

115. The artery that had become occluded resulting in this complication is found most commonly between which vertebral levels?

- **A.** T1 to T5
- **B.** T5 to T10
- **C.** T10 to L2
- **D.** L4 to S2
- **E.** S2 to S4

116. Which of the following neurological findings is commonly associated with this syndrome?

- **A.** Loss of proprioception
- **B.** Loss of pain and temperature sensation
- **C.** Quadriplegia
- **D.** Constipation
- **E.** Loss of vibration sensation

End of set

---

117. During your morning rounds, a 45-year-old male patient you admitted the night before with a small subdural hematoma is found to have new mental status changes. Although a painful sternal rub is applied, the patient fails to open his eyes, proceeds to extend his legs while flexing his upper extremities, and makes a low-pitched moan as his only verbal response. What is this patient's Glasgow Coma Score (GCS)?

- **A.** 3
- **B.** 4
- **C.** 5
- **D.** 6
- **E.** 7

The next two questions (items 118 and 119) correspond to the following vignette.

A 48-year-old male is admitted to the ICU after being found unconscious in a neighborhood park. The patient was intubated while in the emergency department, and he remains on a ventilator with maintenance IV fluids running. You are called emergently to the bedside because the patient has become progressively hypotensive over the last 45 minutes, with a present blood pressure of 78/40 and a heart rate of 130, which is down from 116/64 an hour ago. In addition to giving the patient a fluid bolus, you place a pulmonary artery catheter. The cardiac index is 6.1 L/min/M^2, CVP is 4 mm Hg, PCWP is 10 mm Hg, and SVR is 400 dynes/s/cm^5.

118. What type of shock is this patient experiencing?

- **A.** Septic shock
- **B.** Obstructive shock
- **C.** Hypovolemic shock
- **D.** Neurogenic shock
- **E.** Cardiogenic shock

119. What is the most appropriate next step in the management of this patient?

- **A.** Vasopressin
- **B.** IV fluids
- **C.** Fresh frozen plasma transfusion
- **D.** Dobutamine drip
- **E.** Norepinephrine drip

End of set

The next two questions (items 120 and 121) correspond to the following vignette.

You admit a trauma patient involved in a motorcycle accident who was brought to the emergency department by helicopter in critical condition. The patient has multiple injuries identified on physical exam and with CT scans of his head, chest, abdomen, and pelvis. His injuries include a subdural bleed, two right rib fractures without evidence of a pneumothorax, a traumatic bowel perforation that requires a bowel resection, and a tibial fracture. Following your exploratory laparotomy, the patient was taken to the surgical intensive care unit. You are called 5 hours later by the SICU nurse, who is concerned because the patient has a blood pressure of 82/58 and a heart rate of 116. The nurse gives you the following pulmonary artery numbers: CI of 3.1 L/min/M^2, CVP of 2 mm Hg, PCWP of 9 mm Hg, and SVR of 1600 dynes/s/cm^5.

120. What type of shock is this patient experiencing?

- **A.** Hypovolemic shock
- **B.** Cardiogenic shock
- **C.** Septic shock
- **D.** Neurogenic shock
- **E.** Obstructive shock

121. On admission to the hospital, this patient's hematocrit was 42%. You tell the nurse to check this level, and when you arrive to the SICU you find it to be 22%. The patient remains intubated and continues to follow commands. Where is the patient most likely bleeding to cause a 20 point decline in hematocrit?

A. Pleural cavity
B. Abdominal cavity
C. Retroperitoneal space
D. Intracranial
E. Leg
F. Unidentified injury

End of set

The next two questions (items 122 and 123) correspond to the following vignette.

You are called to the ICU bedside of a 53-year-old female who has been on a ventilator for the last 2 days after undergoing a sigmoid colectomy with diverting colostomy for perforated diverticulitis. The patient remains on IV antibiotics but has been showing signs of sepsis; however, she has not required any vasopressors. Vital signs are BP 102/76, HR 98, RR 20, and T 37.6°C. The ventilator is set on pressure support ventilation, FiO_2 0.50, PIP 14, PEEP 5, and ventilator set rate of 14. The most recent arterial blood gas shows a pH of 7.28, PCO_2 53, PO_2 88, HCO_3 23, and BE –2.

122. What is the proper interpretation of this blood gas reading?

A. Metabolic acidosis
B. Metabolic alkalosis
C. Respiratory acidosis
D. Respiratory alkalosis
E. Combined metabolic and respiratory acidosis

123. How can you best correct this abnormality?

A. Give 2 amps of $NaHCO_3$
B. Increase the FiO_2
C. Increase the respiratory rate
D. Change the IV fluids to 0.9% NS
E. Increase the PIP

End of set

The next two questions (items 124 and 125) correspond to the following vignette.

You are called to evaluate a 3-week-old premature female infant born with a tetralogy of Fallot. The child has recently become distended and is having bilious emesis. The patient's vital signs are stable, and an abdominal film is obtained (Figure 124A).

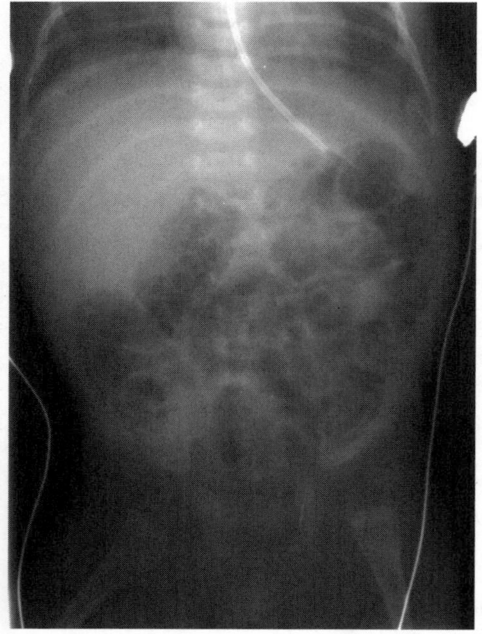

Figure 124A • Image courtesy of the University of Utah School of Medicine, Salt Lake City, Utah.

124. What diagnosis concerns you most at this point?

- **A.** Malrotation
- **B.** Necrotizing enterocolitis
- **C.** Jejunal atresia
- **D.** Meconium ileus
- **E.** Meconium plug syndrome

125. Which of the following is part of the initial management of this condition?

- **A.** Nasogastric decompression
- **B.** Anaerobic antibiotic coverage
- **C.** Placement of a feeding tube
- **D.** Emergent laparotomy
- **E.** Diagnostic laparoscopy

End of set

The next four questions (items 126–129) correspond to the following vignette.

A 37-year-old male is involved in an industrial accident in which he sustains total body surface area burns consisting of 56% of partial- and full-thickness burns. The patient is transferred to your facility, where he undergoes proper resuscitation with Ringer lactate and albumin. After having a feeding tube placed, you need to calculate his daily caloric requirements.

126. What will be his estimated resting energy expenditure?

A. 10 to 20 kcal/kg/day
B. 20 to 30 kcal/kg/day
C. 30 to 40 kcal/kg/day
D. 40 to 50 kcal/kg/day
E. 50 to 60 kcal/kg/day

127. After 2 weeks of enteral feeding, you want to check your patient's nitrogen balance to ensure that he is receiving adequate nutrition. A 24-hour urine nitrogen sample is collected. How do you convert the grams of urinary nitrogen collected to grams of protein?

A. [urinary nitrogen (g) per 24 hours] × 6.25
B. [urinary nitrogen (g) per 24 hours + 4] × 6.25
C. [urinary nitrogen (g) per 24 hours + 8] × 6.25
D. [urinary nitrogen (g) per 24 hours + 4] × 13.5
E. [urinary nitrogen (g) per 24 hours + 8] × 13.5

128. Which of the following complications of overfeeding can be corrected by increasing fat calories as a percentage of nonprotein calories?

A. Increased CO_2 production
B. Hepatic failure
C. Slower recovery
D. Impaired immune system
E. Catheter sepsis

129. In which of the following situations is enteral feeding potentially possible?

A. Severe pancreatitis
B. Short gut syndrome
C. High-output enterocutaneous fistula
D. Prolonged ileus
E. Prolonged intubation

End of set

The next three questions (items 130–132) correspond to the following vignette.

A 23-year-old obese male is brought to the hospital today by ambulance after being involved in a motor vehicle accident the day before. Initially the patient was evaluated and found to have no injuries, and he had been wearing a seat belt. The morning after the accident, the patient's abdomen became acutely tender after eating, at which time he called for an ambulance. Upon arrival to the hospital, the patient is hemodynamically stable but has an acute abdomen. He is taken to the operating room, where you perform an exploratory laparotomy and find an area of small bowel ischemia without significant spillage. The small area of injured bowel is resected and the abdomen is irrigated prior to closing. Nevertheless, you remained concerned about this patient developing a wound infection.

130. How would this patient's level of contamination be classified?

A. Clean
B. Sterile
C. Clean contaminated
D. Contaminated
E. Dirty

131. On postoperative day 2, this patient develops a fever of 38.9°C. You are called by the nursing staff to evaluate the patient, who has otherwise been doing well. What is the most likely cause of fever at this point in his hospital course?

A. Urinary tract infection
B. Atelectasis
C. Medications
D. Intra-abdominal abscess
E. Line infection

132. The patient is slow to progress and remains in the hospital on postoperative day 7. He is febrile and the incision is erythematous. Upon removal of some of the skin staples to check for a suspected wound infection, you note bilious fluid draining from the wound. A diagnosis of enterocutaneous fistula is made. What is the initial step in the treatment of this complication?

A. Percutaneous drainage of abdominal abscess
B. Control of fistula output
C. Initiation of enteral nutrition
D. Exploratory laparotomy
E. IV fluids and electrolyte repletion

End of set

The next two questions (items 133 and 134) correspond to the following vignette.

A 34-year-old male is transported to the ED by firefighters after he sustained minor burns to both lower extremities upon falling near a bonfire. The patient is admitted to the hospital as a trauma/burn case. Initial evaluation shows the patient to be coherent and talking, with the following vital signs: BP 188/82, HR 119, RR 18, and SaO_2 of 100% on 2 liters oxygen. The burns are approximately 14% of total body surface area in size, involving both lower extremities, with the right lower extremity having circumferential full-thickness burns below the knee.

133. Which potential acute injury concerns you most in this patient?

- **A.** Excessive fluid losses from burn wounds
- **B.** Infection of burns
- **C.** Rhabdomyolysis
- **D.** Compartment syndrome
- **E.** Inhalation injury

134. How do you best evaluate for this condition in this patient?

- **A.** Central venous pressure monitoring
- **B.** Urine myoglobin
- **C.** Sputum gram stain and cultures
- **D.** Blood cultures
- **E.** Check compartment pressures

End of set

The next two questions (items 135 and 136) correspond to the following vignette.

A 28-year-old male is seen in the clinic with a 3-day history of crampy abdominal pain accompanied by nausea and vomiting. The patient denies any bowel movements for 3 days and has not passed any gas in 2 days. At age 8, the patient underwent surgical resection of a Wilms' tumor through a midline laparotomy. On exam, his abdomen is grossly distended and very tender with high-pitched bowel sounds. There is a well-healed midline scar and no evidence of any inguinal or incisional hernia. The patient is afebrile, with a HR of 108 and a BP of 114/88. This morning's WBC count is 10,800.

135. What is the next step in this patient's management?

- **A.** Surgical exploration
- **B.** NGT decompression, IV fluid resuscitation, and reevaluation in 24 to 48 hours
- **C.** Abdominal CT scan
- **D.** Colonoscopy
- **E.** Enteroclysis

136. What is the most likely cause of this clinical entity in this patient?

- **A.** Recurrent cancer
- **B.** Intussusception
- **C.** Hernia
- **D.** Adhesions
- **E.** Midgut volvulus

End of set

---

137. A 46-year-old female is in the hospital on postoperative day 3 after undergoing an exploratory laparotomy for a small bowel obstruction. An ischemic bowel was found during the procedure, and a resection with primary anastomosis was performed. The patient continues to have an ileus and over the last 24 hours there has been 625 cc of drainage from the nasogastric tube. The nurse calls you because the patient has spiked a fever of 38.9°C. The physical exam is essentially normal. At this point in this patient's hospital course, you should be suspicious for what process?

A. Wound infection
B. Intra-abdominal abscess
C. Urinary tract infection
D. Deep venous thrombosis
E. Pneumonia

The next two questions (items 138 and 139) correspond to the following vignette.

A 58-year-old female returns to the emergency department 10 days after undergoing a sigmoid colectomy for chronic diverticulitis. The patient's vital signs are as follows: T 102.3°F, HR 123, BP 83/42, RR 28, and SaO_2 of 88% on RA. On physical exam, the abdomen is distended, diffusely tender in the lower quadrants, with no peritoneal signs present. A CBC reveals a WBC count of 23,000. The patient is admitted to the ICU and receives 4 liters of Ringer lactate, but remains hypotensive at 96/47. A central venous catheter is placed and the initial CVP is 5 mm Hg.

138. What is the most likely cause of this patient's hypotension?

A. Myocardial infarction
B. Hypovolemia
C. Pulmonary embolism
D. Spinal shock
E. Sepsis

139. What is the most appropriate treatment once the patient is clinically stable?

A. IV antibiotics and observation
B. Barium enema
C. Surgical exploration
D. CT scan of abdomen and pelvis
E. Oral antibiotics

End of set

---

140. A 62-year-old Native American female patient with a 10-year history of GERD is found to have a 1.4 cm adenocarcinoma limited to the submucosa of the distal esophagus upon routine endoscopy. There is no evidence of lymph node involvement or distant metastasis. The patient undergoes a transhiatal esophagectomy. On postoperative day 7, the patient has a temperature of 39.4°C, but is otherwise stable. Laboratory values reveal a mild leukocytosis. On physical exam, the abdomen is soft, nondistended, and nontender. Breath sounds are decreased in both bases, with some crackles in the left base. The neck incision is erythematous, tender, and indurated, with some cloudy drainage noted. What is the most likely cause of this patient's fever?

A. Superficial wound infection
B. Wound hematoma
C. Pneumonia
D. Anastomotic leak
E. Intra-abdominal abscess

The next two questions (items 141 and 142) correspond to the following vignette.

A 25-year-old female involved in a motor vehicle accident was admitted to your service 4 days ago. The injuries that this patient sustained included facial lacerations and a severely broken left radius and ulna, requiring external fixation by the orthopedic surgery service. Pain control has been difficult for this patient, and she has been slow to ambulate. You are called by the nursing staff to assess the patient due to an abrupt increase in oxygen requirements and complaints of chest pain. Initial impression reveals a patient in mild distress, complaining of chest pain and a feeling of suffocation, which began 30 minutes ago when she returned to bed after ambulating. The patient is presently receiving 4 L of O_2 by nasal cannula with saturations in the low 90s. Your exam reveals the following: Cognition is intact, without focal neurological deficits, tachycardia, and few crackles in the right lung base. The left arm is dressed, and other extremities are warm, without edema. An ECG demonstrates sinus tachycardia, at a rate of 130. The recorded heart rate an hour earlier was 75. Other vital signs are T 37.6°C and BP 124/76. A CXR obtained is unchanged from 2 days ago, which was normal.

141. What test should be ordered next for this patient?

A. CT scan of the thorax
B. Ventilation perfusion lung scan
C. Duplex scanning of lower extremities
D. Pulmonary angiography
E. Transthoracic echocardiogram

142. The test ordered confirms your suspected diagnosis. What treatment should be immediately initiated?

A. β-Blocker, aspirin, and nitroglycerin
B. Lorazepam taper
C. IV fluid bolus
D. Systemic anticoagulation
E. Thoracentesis

End of set

143. After surgically repairing your patient's ruptured abdominal aneurysm, the intubated patient is transferred to the ICU, where massive fluid resuscitation continues. Despite a stable hematocrit, 24 hours postoperatively the patient becomes progressively more oliguric, with elevated peak airway pressures, and tense distention of his abdomen on physical exam. The patient's BP is 110/80 with a HR of 120. What is the best option for this patient at this point?

A. Emergent angiogram to evaluate for possible renal artery damage during AAA repair
B. Abdominal decompression
C. Increase positive end expiratory pressure and give diuretics
D. Transesophageal echo and Swan-Ganz placement
E. Increasing IV fluid rate with an epinephrine drip infusion

The next two questions (items 144 and 145) correspond to the following vignette.

The medical ICU service consults you about a patient with pancreatitis. The patient has no history of alcohol abuse, and a recent ultrasound shows no evidence of gallstones or acute cholecystitis. The patient has been experiencing severe nausea and vomiting and is beginning to have mental status changes. Labs are reviewed: WBC 18,000, hematocrit 32%, amylase 466 U/L, lipase 1176 U/L, serum creatinine 1.2 mg/dL, and calcium 14 mg/dL.

144. What is the proper management of this patient at this time?

A. Start imipenem
B. Start parenteral nutrition
C. Transfuse 2 units packed red blood cells
D. Increase IV fluids to maintain urine output of 80 to 100 cc/h
E. Perform laparoscopic cholecystectomy

145. What medication may be indicated to assist in the emergent management of this condition?

A. Ondansetron
B. Furosemide
C. Ticarcillin/clavulanate
D. Promethazine
E. Phosphate

End of set

The next three questions (items 146–148) correspond to the following vignette.

A 36-year-old female is referred to you for evaluation of periodic abdominal pain that occurs 30 to 40 minutes after eating. The pain and vomiting are most common after she consumes a fatty meal, and the patient reports having symptoms for the last 3 to 4 weeks. A right upper quadrant ultrasound reveals cholelithiasis. You take her to the operating room, where you perform an uncomplicated laparoscopic cholecystectomy. After removing the gallbladder, you open it and find multiple brown stones.

146. Development of brown gallstones is frequently associated with which of the following conditions?

A. Infection
B. Hyperbilirubinemia
C. Cholangiocarcinoma
D. Complete cystic duct obstruction
E. Hypercholesterolemia

147. Which of the following ethnic groups has an increased incidence of brown pigment stone formation?

A. African Americans
B. Caucasians
C. Asians
D. Scandinavians
E. Hispanics

148. Which of the following bacteria most commonly produces the enzyme, bacterial β-d-glucuronidase, that is involved in the formation of brown pigment stones?

A. *Staphylococcus aureus* and *Enterococcus*
B. *Staphylococcus aureus* and *Streptococcus*
C. *Pseudomonas* and *E. coli*
D. *E. coli* and *Bacteroides fragilis*
E. *E. coli* and *Klebsiella*

End of set

The next two questions (items 149 and 150) correspond to the following vignette.

A 32-year-old male presents to your clinic for evaluation of gallstones. The patient describes multiple episodes of biliary colic to you and brings a report of an ultrasound that confirmed the presence of multiple gallstones. You recommend that he undergo a laparoscopic cholecystectomy with an intraoperative cholangiogram. The evening following the cholecystectomy, the patient develops a fever of 40°C. The morning WBC count is elevated to 21,000 and all of the liver function tests are slightly elevated. You start the patient on antibiotics to treat the cholangitis.

149. Which bacteria are most commonly associated with cholangitis?

A. *Enterobacter*
B. *E. coli*
C. *Enterococcus*
D. *Klebsiella*
E. *Proteus*

150. The triad of right upper quadrant pain, fever, and jaundice—commonly known as Charcot's triad—is associated with cholangitis or an active infection in the biliary system. This combination of symptoms can be associated with which two additional symptoms of severe cholangitis?

A. Nausea and elevated WBC
B. Hypertension and chills
C. Mental status changes and hypotension
D. Diarrhea and elevated alkaline phosphatase
E. Oliguria and vomiting

End of set

Block

THREE

Answers and Explanations

Block

THREE

Answer Key

101. E
102. C
103. A
104. C
105. B
106. B
107. B
108. A
109. E
110. D
111. B
112. C
113. C
114. C
115. C
116. B
117. D
118. A
119. B
120. A
121. A
122. C
123. E
124. B
125. A
126. D
127. B
128. A
129. E
130. C
131. B
132. E
133. D
134. E
135. A
136. D
137. C
138. E
139. D
140. D
141. B
142. D
143. B
144. D
145. B
146. A
147. C
148. E
149. B
150. C

101. **E.** Meconium ileus is an obstruction of the distal ileum from inspissated meconium and is often associated with cystic fibrosis. Approximately 10% to 15% of infants with meconium ileus have cystic fibrosis. Meconium ileus presents with failure to pass meconium within 48 hours of birth in conjunction with progressive abdominal distention and bilious emesis. Abdominal films show the classic "soap bubble" appearance in the proximal colon, and a contrast enema shows a microcolon with small plugs of meconium (note the arrows in Figure 101B).

A. Budd-Chiari syndrome is hepatic veno-occlusive disease, mostly seen in adults and not associated with meconium ileus.

B. Down syndrome (trisomy 21) is most often associated with cardiac and renal abnormalities. Associated abdominal abnormalities include imperforate anus, duodenal or jejunal atresia, duodenal or jejunal stenosis, and Hirschsprung's disease.

C. Von Hippel-Lindau syndrome is associated with pancreatic, central nervous system, and renal tumors in adults.

D. Eaton-Lambert syndrome is a paraneoplastic neurologic-myopathic syndrome that presents with symptoms similar to myasthenia gravis.

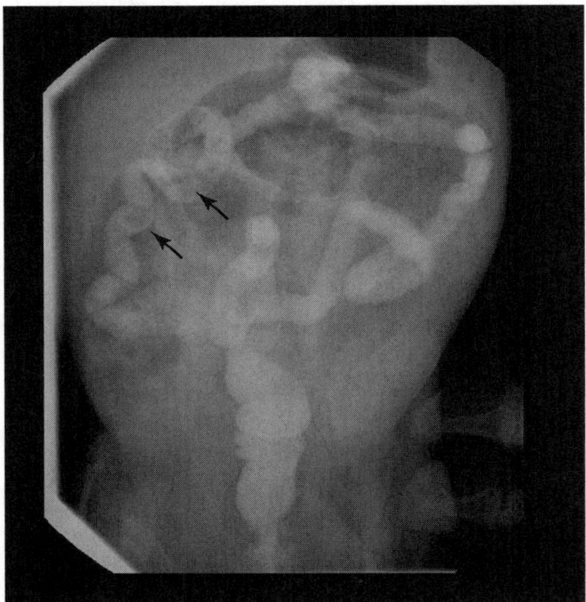

Figure 101B • Image courtesy of the University of Utah School of Medicine, Salt Lake City, Utah.

102. C. Bilious emesis in a newborn should be evaluated immediately to rule out malrotation and midgut volvulus. The "double bubble" sign seen in Figure 102B (note the arrows) is associated with duodenal atresia. Duodenal atresia is frequently associated with other anomalies such as anal atresia, tracheoesophageal fistula with esophageal atresia, and vertebral defects. Duodenal obstruction can be due to a duodenal web, duodenal atresia, duodenal stenosis, or annular pancreas.

A. A midgut volvulus is a surgical emergency due to compromised blood supply to the bowel and increases the risk for developing ischemic bowel. It is part of the differential diagnosis for newborns with bilious emesis, but a "double bubble" sign is virtually pathognomonic for duodenal atresia.

B. Pyloric stenosis presents as rapid, nonbilious projectile vomiting of feeding in infants approximately 6 to 8 weeks of age. It is more common in males than in females (4:1 ratio), and is most common in first-born males.

D. Meconium ileus is a distal ileal obstruction caused by thick, inspissated meconium. It is frequently associated with cystic fibrosis. X-ray findings include dilated loops of bowel and a ground-glass appearance of meconium mixed with air in the right lower quadrant (soap bubble sign).

E. Hirschsprung's disease involves an aganglionic colonic segment with secondary colonic obstruction. It is not associated with bilious emesis.

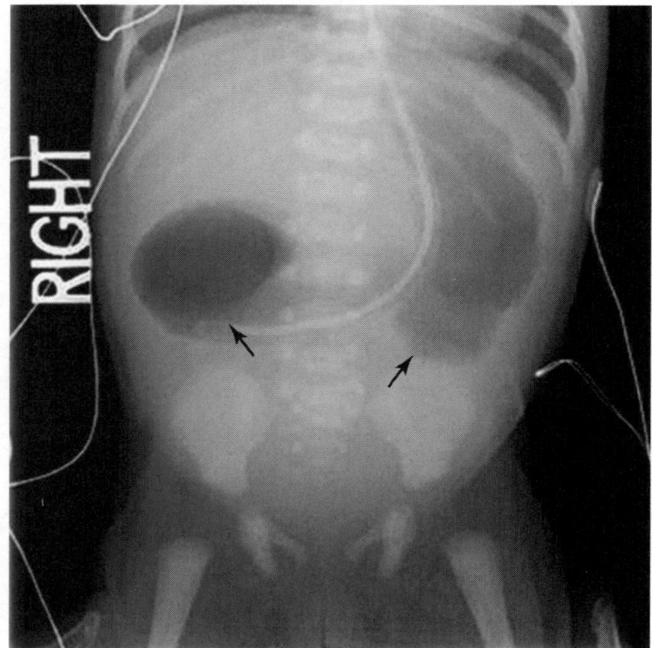

Figure 102B • Image courtesy of the University of Utah School of Medicine, Salt Lake City, Utah.

103. **A.** An anal fissure is a disruption of the anoderm. It most commonly occurs in the posterior midline as a result of forceful dilatation of the anal canal, most often during defecation. Initially it is felt as a tearing pain upon defecation. This pain causes the patient to ignore the urge to defecate, resulting in constipation and further disruption to the anoderm upon defecation. A cycle of pain, poor sphincteric relaxation, and reinjury occurs. The patient presents with pain upon defecation and minimal bleeding noted on tissue with stool. Physical exam by simply separating the buttocks will reveal a tear in the anoderm in the posterior midline.

B. Protrusion of an internal hemorrhoid usually results in anal fullness and discomfort along with bright red blood per rectum. Occasionally, an internal hemorrhoid can prolapse through the anus and incarcerate, requiring surgical intervention. Hemorrhoids can usually be distinguished from a fissure on physical exam.

C. A fistula in ano presents as a draining site on the buttock skin, usually as a complication of an anorectal abscess. It presents with drainage, not extreme pain.

D. Perirectal and anorectal abscesses most often arise from obstruction of an anal gland that subsequently becomes infected and overgrown with bacteria. These glands are located between the internal and external anal sphincters. If the infection tracks down this space toward the skin, an anorectal abscess occurs.

E. Anal condylomas are caused by infection with human papillomavirus (HPV) types 6 and 11. Patients complain of a perianal growth that appears as a cauliflower-like lesion on physical exam. Minimal disease may be treated in the office with bichloracetic acid or podophyllum. Larger lesions may require surgical excision.

104. **C.** Initial treatment with stool softeners, bulking agents, and sitz baths will heal 90% of all anal fissures. A second episode may be treated in the same manner with a 70% success rate.

A. Surgical treatment is reserved for patients who fail conservative management.

B. A 0.2% nitroglycerin topical ointment is an effective treatment, although some studies call its use into question. Side effects may include headaches and tachyphylaxis.

D. Botulinum toxin has been found to be an effective treatment in the healing of anal fissures. However, due to its expense and concerns about paralysis of the anal sphincter, it has not been widely accepted as a therapy for this indication.

E. Patients with this disorder are very uncomfortable and require treatment.

105. **B.** Lateral internal anal sphincterotomy is the procedure of choice after failure to respond to medical management. Patients with fissures of the anus persisting for longer than 1 month as well as patients with chronic, recurring fissures should be considered candidates for surgery. In this procedure, the internal anal sphincter is divided, relieving the spasm that causes the pain and limits the healing. Fecal continence is maintained by the external anal sphincter. This procedure has a success rate exceeding 90%.

A. Although a diverting colostomy would allow the anal fissure to heal, it is a drastic measure and not appropriate in this patient.

C. A low anterior resection is used to treat rectal tumors that are located more than 5 cm from the anal verge.

D. Incision and drainage are more appropriate in the treatment of a perianal abscess.

E. Hemorrhoidectomy would be appropriate for the treatment of hemorrhoids.

106. **B.** This patient has developed severe heart failure and will likely need a transplant to survive. Assist devices are intended as a bridge to transplant. A left ventricular assist device (LVAD) is used for left heart failure, and a right ventricular assist device (RVAD) is used for right heart failure. A biventricular assist device is the best choice in this scenario because the patient has developed bilateral heart failure.

A. The patient's aortic valve is unlikely to be contributing to her condition, and its replacement would not help the situation. The patient is suffering from a severe dilated cardiomyopathy, which will likely be definitively cured only with a heart transplant.

C. A coronary artery bypass graft is performed for ischemic myocardium, which is not the case here.

D. ECMO is used most commonly in children as a means of delivering oxygen to the circulation and removing carbon dioxide in pulmonary or cardiopulmonary failure.

E. This patient's medical management has already been maximized.

107. **B.** An intra-aortic balloon pump decreases afterload by deflating during systole, and by decreasing both the pressure against which the left ventricle must pump and the work of the heart during systole. The balloon inflates during diastole, increasing aortic pressure, which augments coronary and visceral perfusion.

A. A balloon pump deflates during systole.

C. A balloon pump is contraindicated in aortic regurgitation.

D. Use of a balloon pump increases mesenteric flow by inflating during diastole.

E. Although bleeding is always a concern when placing an intra-aortic balloon pump, this alone would not prevent its use.

108. **A.** This patient has pseudo-obstruction (Ogilvie syndrome), which is a paralytic ileus of the large intestine. Painless distention is a common presenting finding. Risk factors include severe blunt trauma, orthopedic trauma or procedures, cardiac disease, acute neurologic disease, and acute metabolic derangements. This condition is dangerous, because the cecum can expand to as much as 10 to 12 cm and possibly perforate.

B, C, D, E. Acute SBO, toxic megacolon, C. *difficile* colitis, and mesenteric ischemia are all possibilities, but are inconsistent with this patient's clinical presentation.

109. **E.** The best initial management of this problem is the correction of metabolic derangements and minimization of narcotic use. When the cecum becomes extremely distended, however, decompression is needed to prevent perforation. Decompression can be accomplished by using neostigmine or by performing a colonoscopy.

A. Exploratory laparotomy is not indicated unless colonic perforation is suspected by clinical exam.

B. Neither antibiotics nor proton pump inhibitors have a role in this situation.

C. It is too early to consider TPN, and its use would not influence the bowel distention.

D. The patient should remain on strict bowel rest until the ileus resolves and should not be started on nasojejunal feedings.

110. **D.** Neostigmine therapy works by preventing destruction of acetylcholine by acetylcholinesterase, and by overcoming the parasympathetic paralytic ileus present. However, neostigmine use carries a risk of life-threatening AV node block, so this patient must be on continuous cardiac monitoring. β-Blocking agents are contraindicated during neostigmine administration. Atropine should be available at the bedside.

A, B, C, E. Chest x-ray, ECG, continuous pulse oximetry, and a baseline ABG are all unnecessary prior to administration of neostigmine. Due to the risks of sudden heart block associated with the administration of neostigmine, continuous cardiac monitoring is the only required treatment.

111. **B.** The most common cause of hemodynamically significant lower GI bleeding is angiodysplasia or an arteriovenous malformation (AVM) within the colon. Overall, the most common source of lower GI bleeding (bright red blood per rectum) is upper GI bleeding with rapid intestinal transit. This condition is often seen in the ICU setting. The quickest and easiest way to diagnose upper GI bleeding is to place a nasogastric tube (NGT).

A. A barium enema is not an indicated test in an emergent situation.

C. Rigid proctoscopy limits visualization to the rectum, which does not allow you to define any colonic sources of bleeding.

D. Colonoscopy is, in most centers, the first diagnostic option after an upper GI bleeding source has been ruled out. It allows the operator to definitively treat a bleeding source once it is located and to mark the area for surgery by using ink injections if needed.

E. Proceeding to the operating room is not indicated until the source of the bleeding has been located. It is difficult to locate an intraluminal source of bleeding in the operating room.

112. **C.** Angiography offers an opportunity for definitive treatment with embolization of the bleeding arteries, but there is the potential for bowel ischemia and infarction after the procedure. The bleeding must be fairly rapid, at least 1 cc/min, to be detected by angiography. For elderly patients with multiple co-morbidities, this is a valuable option due to the increased risk of surgery associated with multiple co-morbidities.

A, B. Bleeding of a small bowel source can be identified with angiography.

D. Cauterization does not affect your ability to visualize the anatomy during angiography.

E. Angiography is a tool used to locate bleeding vessels and define anatomy of the vasculature, but not to diagnose intestinal tumors.

113. **C.** Testicular cancer is the most common solid tumor found in young adult men. Cryptorchidism is the failure of the testicle to descend into the scrotum; it significantly increases the affected individual's risk of testicular cancer. Although cryptorchid testicles should be placed back in the scrotum (orchiopexy), this step does not alter their malignant potential; however, it does facilitate examination and tumor detection.

A. Ninety-five percent of testicular tumors arise from germ cells. These tumors include seminomas, non-seminomas, embryonal cell carcinomas, choriocarcinomas, and teratomas.

B. Human chorionic gonadotropin (hCG) is found in almost 100% of choriocarcinomas, but not seminomas.

D. Seeding of malignant cells can occur along the biopsy tract site. Therefore, orchiectomies should be approached through an inguinal incision.

E. Seminomas are highly sensitive—not insensitive—to radiation therapy.

114. **C.** This patient suffers from anterior cord syndrome, which occurs as a result of ischemia of the spinal cord either from cross-clamping of the aorta or from a low flow state. It is a rare complication of repair of a thoracolumbar aortic aneurysm, or ruptured abdominal aortic aneurysm. When this syndrome is suspected, the most sensitive and specific exam is an MRI of the spinal cord to confirm the diagnosis and delineate the extent of the injury. Figures 114A and 114B are T2 weighted MRI images of the spinal cord. The arrows identify the area damaged by an ischemic event leading to anterior cord syndrome.

A. Electromyography of the lower extremities would be more helpful in determining a progressive neurological loss to the lower extremities, not an acute event.

B. A lumbar puncture should be used in cases of suspected meningitis, which is not the case here.

D. The patient has clinical signs that localize the neurological injury to the spinal cord, not the head.

E. Lumbar myelogram would be helpful in visualizing a mass lesion causing these symptoms, but would be of little use in identifying an injury to the parenchyma of the spinal cord.

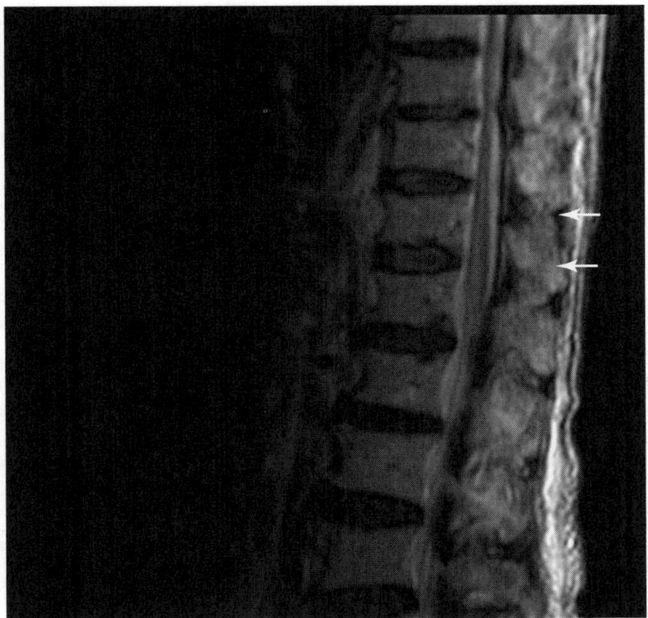

Figure 114A • Image courtesy of the University of Utah School of Medicine, Salt Lake City, Utah.

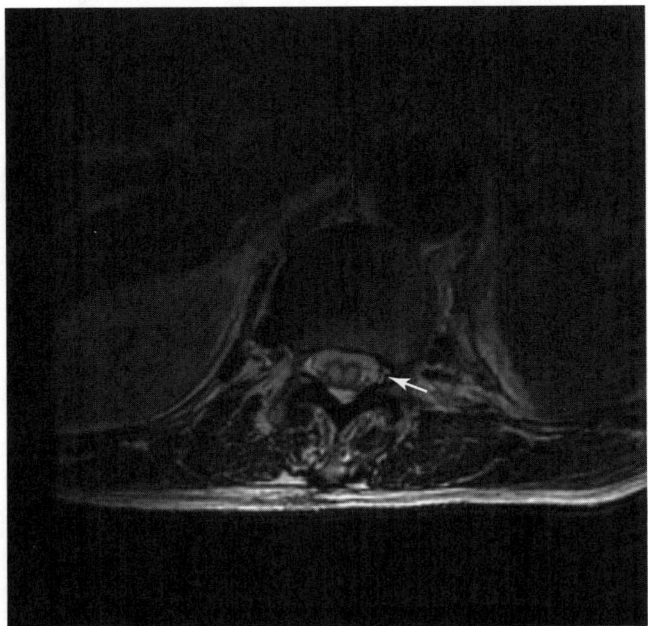

Figure 114B • Image courtesy of the University of Utah School of Medicine, Salt Lake City, Utah.

115. **C.** The great anterior radicular artery (artery of Adamkiewicz) is usually found in the inferior thoracic (T10 to T12) or superior lumbar (L1 to L2) region. It is larger than the other radicular arteries and is of clinical importance because it supplies the major arterial contribution to the anterior spinal artery. This artery provides the main blood supply to the inferior two-thirds of the spinal cord. It is most likely to be damaged or occluded during a thoracolumbar aortic aneurysm repair.

A, B, D, E. These levels do not usually correspond to the origin of the great anterior radicular artery.

116. **B.** The anterior spinal artery supplies the anterior two-thirds of the spinal cord with blood via the sulcal artery. An occlusion of the great anterior radicular artery (artery of Adamkiewicz) causes an infarction of the anterior two-thirds of the spinal cord, sparing the posterior one-third that is supplied by the posterior spinal artery. Loss of pain and temperature sensation occurs because of infarction of the lateral spinothalamic tracts, which carry pain and temperature sensation to the thalamus.

A. The dorsal columns, which carry sensory fibers for proprioception, remain intact.

C. Infarction of the lateral and ventral corticospinal tracts causes paralysis below the affected level, usually resulting in paraplegia, not quadriplegia.

D. Damage associated with the conus medullaris or the inferior-most portion of the spinal cord will cause loss of bowel and bladder control, not constipation.

E. Vibration is sensed via fibers in the dorsal columns, which remain intact.

117. **D.** The Glasgow Coma Scale is a scoring tool used to quantify level of consciousness; it is used to initially assess prognosis in patients with a head injury. The grading system evaluates the best verbal, motor, and ocular responses (Table 117). A coma is usually seen with a score less than 8. This patient's scores are as follows: eye opening—does not open eyes (1); motor response—decorticate posture (3); and verbal response—incomprehensible sounds (2).

A, B, C, E. These options all give incorrect calculations for the GCS.

TABLE 117 Glasgow Coma Grading System

Assessment	Score
Eye opening	4: Opens spontaneously 3: Opens to voice (command) 2: Opens to painful stimulus 1: Does not open eyes
Motor response	6: Obeys commands 5: Localizes painful stimulus 4: Withdraws from pain 3: Decorticate posture 2: Decerebrate posture 1: No movement
Verbal response	5: Appropriate and oriented 4: Confused 3: Inappropriate words 2: Incomprehensible sounds 1: No sounds

118. **A.** This patient is demonstrating symptoms of septic shock. The low systemic vascular resistance combined with an elevated cardiac index is indicative of septic shock. Septic shock is characterized by microvascular permeability mediated by the cytokines TNF-α and IL-1, reactive oxygen radicals, vasoactive peptides, complement, and platelet-activating factor. This cascade of events leads to decreased intravascular volume and third-space fluid losses. Treatment of septic shock is directed at adequate fluid resuscitation followed by vasopressors as needed.

B. Obstructive shock is seen in conditions such as tension pneumothorax and cardiac tamponade. In this type of shock, the PCWP, CVP, and SVR values would he higher.

C. Hypovolemic shock is caused by significant intravascular volume loss, such as with blood loss during trauma or surgery. In this scenario, the CVP and PCWP values would be low and the SVR value would be high.

D. Neurogenic shock is seen with spinal cord injury or anesthetic blocks. Diagnosis is made based on history and physical exam, which shows decreased blood pressure with a paradoxically low pulse rate.

E. Cardiogenic shock is seen with cardiac events that cause depressed cardiac function, such as in a myocardial infarction or with tamponade. In this type of shock, there would be a low CI value, and high CVP and PCWP values.

119. **B.** Prior to starting any type of vasoactive agent, it is vital to ensure that the patient is intravascularly fluid resuscitated. With a CVP of 4 mm Hg and a PCWP of 10 mm Hg, it is appropriate to give this patient more fluid or volume to increase the intravascular volume.

A. Vasopressin increases the cAMP level, which subsequently increases water permeability at the renal tubules. Its use is becoming more common in the management of sepsis. This patient needs adequate fluid resuscitation before starting a vasoactive agent.

C. A fresh frozen plasma transfusion is not indicated in this case, as the patient is not coagulopathic. While he does need volume, it is safest to start with crystalloid fluids.

D. Dobutamine is a vasoactive agent that is primarily a β-agonist. As such, it increases myocardial contractility but does not produce peripheral vasoconstriction.

E. Norepinephrine is the drug of choice in septic shock, but only after the patient is fluid resuscitated. Its potent α-agonist activity provides peripheral vasoconstriction to counteract the global inflammatory response associated with septic shock.

120. **A.** In this scenario, the patient's cardiac index is normal and the systemic vascular resistance is compensating for his being intravascularly volume depleted or hypovolemic. The CVP and PCWP values are both low, so the patient needs volume, starting with crystalloid and following with blood products as needed.

B, C, D, E. See the explanation for question 118 for more detail.

121. **A.** This patient is exhibiting hypovolemic shock and had a 20 point drop in his hematocrit. There are multiple areas in which a trauma patient may bleed, including the pleural space (rib fractures, great vessel injuries), abdomen (solid organ or great vessel injuries), retroperitoneal space (kidneys, pelvis), legs (femur fractures, not lower leg fractures), or bleeding out exteriorly. The pleural cavity is the most likely place in which this patient would be bleeding, as a result of his rib fractures and likely associated intercostal vessel injuries.

B. Abdominal cavity bleeding is likely from the liver, spleen, or other vessel injuries. There were no solid organ injuries by CT, and a bowel perforation would be less likely to cause this type of hematocrit drop.

C. The retroperitoneal space is a possible source of bleeding, as with pelvis fractures or renal injuries. However, this patient did not have any identified retroperitoneal injuries by CT scan or during bowel resection.

D. It is very unlikely that an individual could bleed enough into his or her head that the hematocrit level would change by 20 points. This patient is alert and following commands, which would also argue against a head bleed.

E. While a patient with a femur fracture can bleed a large amount into the thigh, this would be much less likely with below-the-knee fractures.

F. Unidentified injuries are always possible and should not be forgotten.

122. **C.** This patient has a respiratory acidosis due to underventilation. The elevated PCO_2 of 53 properly accounts for the acidemia. For every unit increase of PCO_2 that occurs, the pH will fall by 0.8. Thus, when you correct the pH for a PCO_2 of 53 to a the pH for a PCO_2 of 40, the pH would reflectively show an increase to 7.38, which is normal. From this result, you can conclude that the acidosis is due to underventilation.

A, E. With a base excess of –2 and an HCO_3 of 23, it is safe to say that this patient does not have metabolic acidosis.

B, D. With a pH less than 7.4, the patient is acidotic, not alkalotic.

123. **E.** When a patient is experiencing retained CO_2, ventilation needs to be improved. This is accomplished by increasing the minute ventilation, which entails increasing the respiratory rate or increasing the tidal volume. This patient is already over-breathing to a rate of 20 the ventilator set rate of 14, so increasing the rate would not be helpful. The tidal volume can be increased by raising the peak inspiratory pressure (PIP) to improve ventilation status.

A. Giving sodium bicarbonate ($NaHCO_3$) is helpful in a metabolic acidosis situation to increase the pH. It is not indicated in respiratory acidosis.

B. Increasing the FiO_2 would help to increase the oxygenation, but it would not improve the minute ventilation.

C. The patient is over-breathing the set ventilator rate, and a further increase in the rate would not change her minute ventilation. Increasing the PIP, in this case, would increase the minute ventilation.

D. Changing the IV fluids to normal saline (NS) would not change the overall situation.

124. **B.** Bilious emesis in a newborn is considered a surgical emergency and needs to be evaluated immediately. The x-ray in Figure 124B (see the arrow) shows extensive pneumatosis intestinalis in the descending colon. This finding is concerning for necrotizing enterocolitis (NEC). The etiology of NEC is unknown, but is believed to be associated with ischemic intestine damage and bacterial colonization.

A. Three-fourths of patients with malrotation present with obstruction in infancy due to Ladd's bands (adhesions) or volvulus around the superior mesenteric vessels. Newborns with pneumatosis intestinalis are more likely to have NEC.

C. Jejunal atresia presents with bilious vomiting, but not pneumatosis intestinalis as seen on the abdominal film for this patient.

D. Meconium ileus occurs in 10% to 20% of infants with cystic fibrosis. By history, those babies fail to pass meconium and abdominal films show a "soap bubble" sign in the right lower quadrant. Nonoperative treatment is successful in 60% to 70% of cases.

E. Neonatal small left colon syndrome (meconium plug syndrome) is due to a narrow left colon with proximal dilation of the transverse and right colon on plain abdominal films.

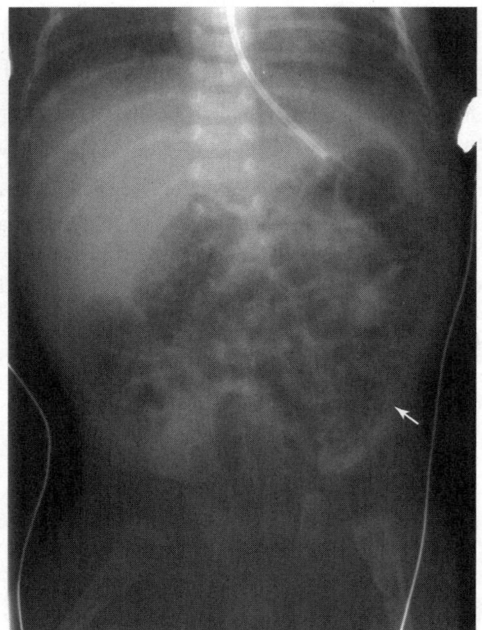

Figure 124B • Image courtesy of the University of Utah School of Medicine, Salt Lake City, Utah.

125. **A.** The pathophysiology of necrotizing enterocolitis (NEC) has been somewhat controversial. Some authors suggest it is related to hypoxic stress during delivery, while more recent studies relate it to infectious causes in a compromised host with immature immune and gut barrier defenses. Proper initial management of NEC includes nasogastric decompression, broad-spectrum antibiotics, bowel rest with TPN, and IV hydration. Once a perforation has occurred and free air is seen on an x-ray, the patient needs an exploratory laparotomy.

B. While anaerobic antibiotic coverage is necessary, broad-spectrum coverage is the most appropriate choice (gram-positive, gram-negative, and anaerobic coverage).

C. Strict bowel rest is necessary for management of NEC. TPN is appropriate for nutritional support.

D. Emergent laparotomy is necessary if the infant has a perforated bowel. Otherwise, it is not part of the initial management.

E. Laparoscopy has no role in the management of NEC.

126. **D.** The caloric requirements of an injured person increase substantially, depending on the severity of the injury. An average individual requires an REE of 30 to 40 kcal/kg/day. Severely stressed individuals, as in this scenario, require 40 to 50 kcal/kg/day.

A, B. Even for a healthy individual, 10 to 30 kcal/kg/day is not adequate.

C. The requirement for maintenance of weight in a nonstressed individual is 30–40 kcal/kg/day.

E. Even for a severely stressed individual, 50 to 60 kcal/kg/day is too many calories.

127. **B.** By measuring the nitrogen balance, nitrogen synthesis and breakdown can be evaluated. Nitrogen intake is the amount of protein taken in, and the output is the total of all excretions and secretions. The urinary urea nitrogen is converted to grams of protein by the following equation: [urinary nitrogen (g) per 24 hours + 4] × 6.25. A correction factor of 4 is added to account for the losses in stool.

A, C, D, E. These are all incorrect formulas.

128. **A.** Increased CO_2 production is a direct result of overfeeding and can be reduced by increasing the percentage of fat calories consumed relative to total calories.

B. Hepatic failure is usually part of the picture for multiple organ dysfunction due to sepsis.

C, D. Overfeeding can cause prolonged recovery and impaired immune response, but these problems will not necessarily be corrected with consumption of an increased percentage of fat calories.

E. Central line sepsis is not directly related to the percentage of fat calories consumed.

129. **E.** Whenever a patient is able to feed using the GI tract, this approach is the method of choice. Nasojejunal tube feedings should be started for patients without conditions that would preclude use of enteral feeding, such as patients with prolonged intubation.

A, B, C, D. Parenteral nutrition is required in a number of clinical scenarios, including in the following situations: severe pancreatitis, where strict bowel rest is necessary; short gut syndrome, due to inadequate bowel length for enteral feeding absorption; a high output enterocutaneous fistula, to decrease secretions and output, thereby allowing the fistula to close; and a prolonged ileus, which precludes enteral feeding until the source of the problem is treated.

130. **C.** A small bowel resection with minimal, contained spillage is considered to be a clean contaminated operative case. Wound infection rates are associated with the level of contamination seen during the surgical case. In a clean contaminated case (GI or respiratory tract entered without significant spillage), a 5% to 8% wound infection rate is seen.

A. A clean case, such as a breast biopsy, has a 1% to 3% rate of wound infection.

B. There is no such classification as a sterile case.

D. A contaminated case, such as a colon injury with bowel spillage, has a 10% to 15% rate of wound infection.

E. A 15% to 40% wound infection rate is seen in a dirty or infected case, such as an intra-abdominal abscess from a colonic anastomosis leak.

131. **B.** Many conditions may cause a postoperative fever. A commonly used mnemonic is the 5 W's: wind, water, wound, walking, and weird drugs. On postoperative day 2, it is less likely that a patient would have pneumonia, a wound infection, or a urinary tract infection. The most common cause of an "early" postoperative fever is atelectasis.

A. Indwelling Foley catheters are foreign bodies and predispose patients to develop urinary tract infections. Postoperative day 2 would be early for a UTI to emerge, but this possibility is easily checked by obtaining a urinalysis.

C. Some medications may induce a fever and should be taken into consideration when making the diagnosis. The vast majority of fevers (approximately 90%) that occur within the first 48 hours, however, are secondary to atelectasis.

D. An intra-abdominal abscess is always a consideration in a surgical case that is considered a contaminated case, but usually the presentation is closer to postoperative day 5.

E. A central line is a foreign body that can easily cause an infection, but a line placed under sterile conditions is unlikely to be the cause of infection so early in the postoperative course.

132. **E.** The initial priority in patients with an enterocutaneous fistula (ECF) is fluid resuscitation and repletion of electrolytes. The difficulty of this task depends on the location of the fistula and the amount of output present. Proximal fistulas usually have a higher output with more electrolyte irregularities. It is imperative to aggressively treat these patients, as their electrolyte levels can rapidly become depleted.

A. After fluid resuscitation the abdomen should eventually be studied by CT scan, looking for the presence of abscesses. If present, they should be drained percutaneously. Ongoing infections limit spontaneous closure of the fistula and increase the risk of death.

B. Control of the fistula entails protecting the skin from enteric contents and assisting in fluid replacement by accurate measurement of output.

C. It is important to begin nutritional support early in the treatment of ECF. Preventing malnutrition decreases the septic mortality and increases the likelihood of spontaneous closure.

D. The decision to perform an exploratory laparotomy is a difficult one in treating patients with an ECF. After fluid resuscitation, this procedure should be performed in patients who continue to have sepsis and a worsening course despite maximal support. In stable patients without ongoing signs of sepsis, it should be done after the patient is nutritionally stable, free from infection, and the fistula has not closed despite maximum non-surgical measures.

133. **D.** Whenever a patient sustains burns that are circumferential in nature on an extremity, you must be concerned about compartment syndrome. It is important to check baseline compartment pressures and follow them serially. Escharotomies should be performed as needed for increasing compartment pressures above 30 mm Hg. This procedure releases the pressure within the compartment and reestablishes blood flow distal to the injury.

A. With every burn injury, concern arises regarding significant fluid losses. Fluid resuscitation is based on standard burn fluid calculations, which should address fluid issues. There is no reason to suspect "excessive" losses beyond those based on standard calculations.

B. Infection of burns is a significant complication, but would not occur in the acute injury situation.

C. Rhabdomyolysis occurs in severe crush injuries or anytime muscle is severely damaged. It is unlikely in a 14% TBSA burn.

E. Inhalation injuries occur most often in closed-space fires (indoors) and should be considered with patients who are symptomatic in terms of respiratory distress. Signs and symptoms can include carbonaceous sputum; burns near the nose, mouth, and face; raspy voice; and hoarseness.

134. **E.** The best way to evaluate for compartment syndrome in an involved area is to evaluate the pressures in the compartment. Elevated compartment pressures in the presence of hypoperfusion are diagnostic for compartment syndrome.

A. CVP measurement is used to evaluate a patient's fluid status.

B. Urine myoglobin measurement is used to evaluate for rhabdomyolysis.

C. Sputum cultures are used to evaluate for pneumonia.

D. Blood cultures are unlikely to be helpful in the acute injury setting.

135. **A.** This patient has a complete small bowel obstruction. The most common presentation includes abdominal distention, diffuse pain, persistent nausea and vomiting, and decreased flatus or bowel movements. It is important to differentiate between a complete versus partial obstruction. Complete obstruction is accompanied by obstipation, or the failure to pass gas or stool within the last 12 hours. Abdominal films usually demonstrate a paucity of gas within the colon and rectum. Complete obstruction is an absolute indication for surgery. This patient complains of obstipation for 2 days. Exploratory laparotomy is warranted to correct the underlying cause of obstruction.

B. Partial obstruction can be accompanied by flatus or diarrhea as well as colonic or rectal gas on abdominal plain films. In both cases, plain abdominal films will demonstrate multiple air-fluid levels and dilated loops of small bowel. Partial small bowel obstructions are usually seen in patients with previous abdominal surgery, which results in adhesion formation. Nonoperative management consists of NPO status, NGT decompression, IV hydration, electrolyte repletion, and close observation. Failure to resolve the obstruction within 48 hours or any change in stability or increased tenderness noted on abdominal exam warrants surgical intervention.

C. An abdominal CT scan may demonstrate a transition point, but it would not change the immediate treatment plan in this case.

D. A colonoscopy would not allow you to visualize the small bowel and would not be helpful.

E. An enteroclysis is the study of choice to localize the obstructed area, but it would not change the initial management of this patient.

136. **D.** The most common causes of small bowel obstruction in the United States are adhesions, hernias, and tumors (in that order). Incarceration of a hernia (femoral, inguinal, or ventral) is the second most common cause of SBO. Tumors may result in occlusion of the bowel lumen or intussusception if the tumor is intrinsic and twisting or entrapment of the small bowel by extrinsic tumors. Intussusception is a possibility, especially in children, but is infrequent in adults.

A, B, C, E. These options are all causes of small bowel obstructions, with adhesions being by far the most common cause in a patient with previous abdominal surgery.

137. **C.** Urinary tract infections typically occur after postoperative day number 3 and are usually accompanied by dysuria and low-grade fever. Diagnosis is made with urinalysis and confirmed by urine cultures. Discontinuation of the Foley catheter and antibiotic therapy are usually sufficient treatment.

A. A wound infection is easily diagnosed by erythema, warmth, tenderness on physical exam, and fever. This patient's physical exam was normal. Treatment would consist of opening the wound and packing it with moist gauze until the wound heals.

B. Intra-abdominal abscesses generally occur 7 to 10 days after surgery. Patients will have complaints of fever, abdominal pain, and abdominal distention with food intolerance. A leukocytosis is usually present. Abdominal and pelvis CT scan is used to diagnose abscesses. If an abscess is identified by CT, it can often be drained percutaneously.

D. Surgery significantly increases the risk for developing a deep vein thrombosis (DVT), due to prolonged stasis of blood during surgery and shortly thereafter. Patients with DVT will often present with fevers early in their course; for that reason, it is important to be aware of the possibility of thrombus formation. Calf, thigh tenderness, and hypoxia with chest pain should also be evaluated for pulmonary embolus from a DVT.

E. Pneumonia often presents with productive cough, fever, tachypnea, decreased breath sounds on auscultation, and dullness to percussion. Management includes antibiotics and aggressive pulmonary toilet. The overall mortality rate from post-operative pneumonia is 20% to 40%.

138. **E.** This patient presents with clinical evidence of shock. Given her recent history, it is very likely that she has an intra-abdominal abscess leading to septic shock. Sepsis results in the release of circulating cytokines during the inflammatory response, causing fever, leukocytosis, and loss of systemic vascular resistance resulting in hypotension refractory to fluid resuscitation.

A, C. Cardiogenic shock results from depressed cardiac function. It may occur secondary to myocardial infarction, pulmonary embolus, arrhythmias, cardiac tamponade, pneumothorax, and toxic doses of medication. This type of shock and its potential causes need to be kept in mind particularly with elderly patients, but this scenario is more consistent with septic shock symptoms.

B. While septic shock patients experience a relative hypovolemia due to the increased third spacing fluid and decreased vascular tone, the underlying process is a global inflammatory response that causes microvascular leaking of intravascular fluid into the interstitium. Fluid resuscitation alone will not always correct the hypotension due to the loss of systemic vascular tone; consequently, vasopressors may be needed.

D. Damage to the cervical spinal cord may result in loss of autonomic innervation, causing depressed myocardial function as well as loss of vascular tone. This type of shock occurs with a history of trauma and would be unlikely in this scenario. It is usually treated with fluid resuscitation and dopamine.

139. **D.** Most septic patients need management in an intensive care setting including central venous access and invasive hemodynamic monitoring. Once the patient has been adequately stabilized with fluids and vasoactive agents, if necessary, the underlying cause of the sepsis needs to be identified and treated. With this patient's recent clinical history, it is likely that she has an intra-abdominal abscess. This problem can best be diagnosed by a CT scan of the abdomen and pelvis.

A. While IV antibiotics are necessary to treat sepsis, an intra-abdominal abscess will not respond to administration of antibiotics alone. Instead, it will require drainage as well, which can be done either percutaneously or surgically.

B. A barium enema helps define the intraluminal anatomy of the bowel; it will not give a picture of an intra-abdominal process.

C. Surgical exploration is necessary if the abscess cannot be adequately drained percutaneously or if the patient has ongoing contamination from an anastomotic leak that fails to close.

E. Oral antibiotics alone are an inadequate treatment. Drainage of the abscess and IV antibiotics are needed.

140. **D.** A transhiatal esophagectomy consists of an abdominal incision with mobilization of the stomach and dissection of the esophagus up to the level of the neck. A left cervical incision is made, and the remainder of the esophagus is mobilized. The esophagus is then removed and an esophagogastric anastomosis is created in the neck. An anastomotic leak occurs in approximately 10% of all patients who undergo esophagectomy with esophagogastrectomy. The risk of a leak is higher with a cervical anastomosis than with an intrathoracic anastomosis. However, the mortality from a cervical anastomotic leak is significantly lower than that associated with an intrathoracic leak. Symptoms of a leak usually appear 5 to 10 days postoperatively and consist of fever, leukocytosis, subcutaneous crepitus, erythema, and wound drainage. If this problem is suspected, the cervical wound should be opened widely and drained. The wound is then packed with dry gauze. Almost all cervical leaks heal with conservative management. One-third of these complications subsequently develop strictures, requiring repeat dilatation.

A. Although this scenario describes a classic wound infection, in patients undergoing a cervical esophagogastric anastomosis, the description would represent an anastomotic leak until proven otherwise.

B. Hematoma, while included in the differential diagnosis, should not be considered first in this scenario.

C, E. Although both of these complications are important in the differential diagnosis of postoperative fever, this presentation with cervical wound changes is most consistent with an anastomotic leak.

141. **B.** Polytrauma patients are at an increased risk of deep vein thrombosis (DVT), and a pulmonary embolus (PE) is the most severe complication of a DVT. Because of this risk, aggressive DVT prophylaxis along with early ambulation should be started in all high-risk patients. The most common symptoms of a PE include dyspnea, chest pain, and a cough. Increased oxygen requirements, tachypnea, and tachycardia are often present when examining a suspected patient with a PE. Given that these signs and symptoms are associated with other cardiopulmonary disorders, it is imperative that you obtain further tests. The ventilation-perfusion lung scan is the pivotal study in hemodynamically stable patients suspected of having a PE. It is safe, noninvasive, and widely available. A normal perfusion scan excludes the diagnosis of PE, whereas a scan with perfusion defects and normal ventilation is highly suggestive of a PE. An indeterminate scan should be followed by a more specific test such as a CT angiogram.

A. CT angiograms of the thorax are becoming increasingly more popular in the diagnosis of a pulmonary embolus. Figure 141 shows a large clot in the right pulmonary artery (note the arrow). A simple CT of the thorax would not be of any diagnostic value in this case.

C. Duplex scanning of the lower extremities is used to evaluate for DVT, but it cannot diagnose a pulmonary embolism. It may be an appropriate study in patients with signs of a PE and simultaneous signs of a DVT. In this case, the patient does not demonstrate symptoms of a DVT.

D. Pulmonary angiography is the most sensitive and specific test in diagnosing a pulmonary embolus, but it is invasive and expensive and has been replaced by CT angiograms in many instances.

E. A transthoracic echocardiogram may be obtained in a critically ill or hemodynamically unstable patient. Right heart dysfunction is usually identified by right ventricular dilation, or aberrant motion of the interventricular septum. Transesophageal studies can visualize thrombi within the pulmonary trunk.

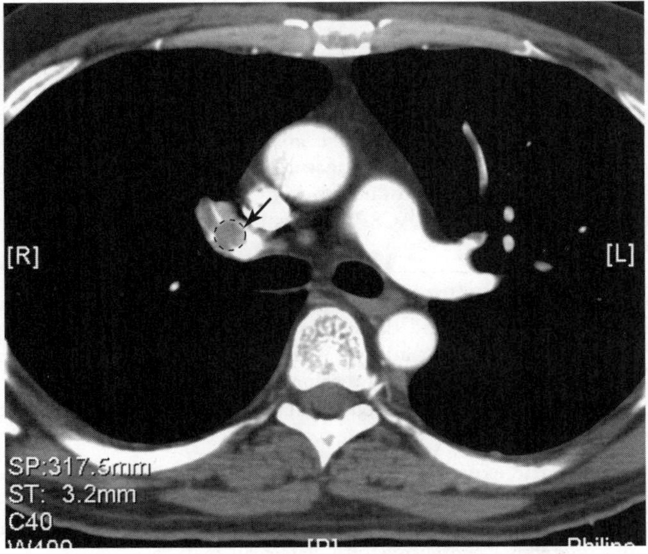

Figure 141 • Image courtesy of the University of Utah School of Medicine, Salt Lake City, Utah.

142. **D.** This patient should be started on systemic heparinization immediately. Once a therapeutic range is obtained and the patient can tolerate oral medications, she should be switched over to warfarin, with the heparin being continued until the PT/INR is therapeutic. Oral anticoagulation is then continued for 3 to 6 months.

A. This choice is the appropriate initial treatment for a patient you suspect of having a myocardial infarction.

B. A lorazepam (Ativan) taper should be initiated in patients suspected of suffering from acute alcohol withdrawal.

C. An IV fluid bolus would be appropriate in the treatment of a patient with hypovolemic shock.

E. A thoracentesis would be indicated in a patient with respiratory embarrassment secondary to a significant pleural effusion.

143. **B.** This case is a classic presentation of abdominal compartment syndrome (ACS) after a repair of a ruptured AAA. ACS may be seen after massive fluid resuscitation as encountered in conjunction with emergent repairs of a ruptured AAA, abdominal trauma, pancreatitis, severe intra-abdominal infections, and severe burns. Increased intra-abdominal pressure results in renal venous compression and increased pressure in the renal parenchyma, which can lead to oliguria. Alteration in microvascular permeability leads to a progressive increase in intra-abdominal pressure and subsequently decreased cardiac output due to decreased venous return and increased systemic vascular resistance. The transmission of the intra-abdominal hypertension to the chest reduces ventilatory compliance and necessitates increased airway pressures to maintain adequate ventilation and oxygenation. The diagnosis of ACS is based on recognition of the clinical syndrome of tense abdominal distention, signs of decreased cardiac output, elevated airway pressures, and oliguria. Intra-abdominal pressure (IAP) is measured indirectly and easily by measuring the bladder pressure using a Foley catheter and pressure transducer system, with pressures greater than 15 mm Hg being consistent with ACS. Treatment of ACS is surgical abdominal decompression.

A. The majority of abdominal aortic aneurysms have a "neck" of normal aorta between the renal artery ostia and the beginning of the aneurysm, allowing for their repair without renal vascular injury. While oliguria may be related to either renal vascular injury or prolonged hypotension leading to acute tubular necrosis (ATN), in this case oliguria and increased ventilatory pressures are the most overt clinical ramifications of ACS.

C. Increased positive end expiratory pressure (PEEP) may be needed to temporarily support ventilation, but it will not treat—and may actually exacerbate—the increased intra-abdominal pressure found in ACS. Diuretics should not be given to a patient who is relatively hypotensive with classic signs of ACS.

D. Transesophageal echo (TEE) and Swan-Ganz (SG) pressure measurements would show decreased cardiac output due to decreased venous return and artificially elevated left and right heart pressures secondary to increased intrathoracic pressures. In ACS, the TEE and SG catheter measurements would show the effects of increased intra-abdominal pressure rather than primary cardiac dysfunction. The patient would still require abdominal decompression, given the information derived from the TEE and SG placement.

E. Increasing the amount of intravenous fluids may potentiate the ACS rather than relieve the problem. Added vasoactive support may transiently improve the hemodynamic status but it will not improve renal perfusion or urine output in the clinical condition of ACS described.

144. **D.** The two most common causes of pancreatitis are alcohol and gallstones. This patient does not show any evidence of gallstones on the ultrasound and has no history of alcohol abuse. Among the other causes of pancreatitis is hypercalcemia. In this case, the patient's calcium level is 14 mg/dL. With the onset of mental status changes, aggressive therapy must be started. Aggressive fluid resuscitation should be instituted and monitored by following the patient's urine output.

A. There is no indication for antibiotic therapy at this time.

B. While total parenteral nutrition (TPN) may be needed if the pancreatitis does not resolve, it is not indicated at this time.

C. There is no need for blood transfusion with a hematocrit of 32% and no evidence of bleeding.

E. A cholecystectomy is not indicated in a patient with a negative US for gallstones or without acute cholecystitis.

145. **B.** Once the patient is adequately hydrated, administration of a loop diuretic such as furosemide (Lasix) promotes calcium excretion. Other medications that may be used include steroids, mithramycin, and calcitonin. Renal dialysis may be required if medication proves ineffective or if the situation is critical.

A, D. Antiemetics do not have a role in the management of hypercalcemia.

C. Antibiotics do not have a role in calcium reduction.

E. Phosphate does not have a role in the management of hypercalcemia.

146. **A.** Gallstones are composed of bile salts, cholesterol, and lecithin. They are typically classified as either cholesterol or pigmented stones (black or brown). The cholesterol stones account for 75% of all gallstones, while the black and brown pigmented stones account for 20% and 5%, respectively. Brown stones are frequently associated with infection and are typically found in Asian patients. Primary common duct stones are frequently brown gallstones.

B. Hyperbilirubinemia associated with gallstones occurs when the hepatic duct or common duct becomes obstructed. Brown stones are not directly related to increased levels of bilirubin.

C. There is no increase in the incidence of cholangiocarcinoma with brown gallstones.

D. Cystic duct obstruction occurs with any type of gallstone, resulting in pain and nausea following consumption of a fatty meal. There is no increase in the incidence of cystic duct obstruction with brown stones.

E. Brown gallstones are not associated with hypercholesterolemia.

147. **C.** Asians have a higher incidence of developing brown gallstones than non-Asian individuals. The reasons for this propensity are not clearly understood.

A, B, D, E. These ethnic groups are not associated with an increased incidence of brown gallstones.

148. **E.** The enzyme β-d-glucuronidase drives the hydrolysis of bilirubin glucuronide into free bilirubin and glucuronic acid. The free unconjugated bilirubin can then combine with the calcium in bile to form pigmented stones. This enzyme is produced by *E. coli* and *Klebsiella*, both enteric bacteria commonly found in bile.

A. *Enterococcus* is an enteric bacterium that is found in bile and does not produce the enzyme β-d-glucuronidase. *Staphylococcus aureus* is common skin flora; it is not usually found in bile.

B. *Staphylococcus* and *Streptococcus* are not usually found in bile and do not produce the enzyme β-d-glucuronidase.

C, D. *E. coli* is commonly found in bile and produces the enzyme β-d-glucuronidase. *Pseudomonas* and *Bacteroides fragilis* do not produce the enzyme and are not commonly found in bile.

149. **B.** Numerous bacteria are associated with cholangitis. Not surprisingly, they are most commonly related to normal gut flora. *E. coli* is the most common bacteria associated with cholangitis at 35%, followed by *Enterococcus* (16%), *Klebsiella* (14%), *Proteus* (12%), *Pseudomonas* (9%), and *Enterobacter* (5%).

A, C, D, E. See the explanation for B.

150. **C.** Mental status changes and hypotension are grave signs of biliary sepsis and demand urgent treatment to decompress the biliary tree. This grouping is termed Reynolds' pentad.

A. Nausea and an increased WBC count may occur in severe cholangitis, but not as a part of Reynolds' pentad.

B. Hypotension—not hypertension—is a sign of biliary sepsis and severe cholangitis.

D. Diarrhea and elevated alkaline phosphatase may be seen, but they do not complete the pentad of symptoms.

E. Oliguria and vomiting may be seen, but they do not complete the pentad of symptoms.

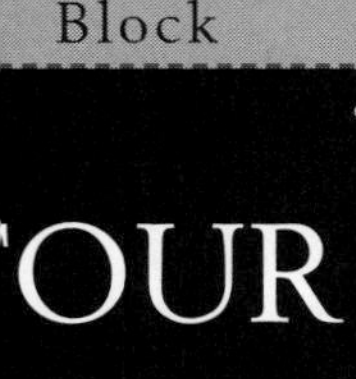

Questions

Setting 4: Emergency Department

Generally, patients encountered here are seeking urgent care; most are not known to you. A full range of social services is available, including rape crisis intervention, family support, child protective services, domestic violence support, psychiatric services, and security assistance backed up by local police. Complete laboratory and radiology services are available.

The next three questions (items 151–153) correspond to the following vignette.

A 66-year-old male presents to the emergency room with acute onset of right leg pain. The patient states that the pain started 2 hours ago and is unrelenting, and he claims that the leg is "tingling." On your examination, it looks pale and feels cold to touch, and there are no Doppler-able pedal signals.

151. What is the most appropriate next step in the management of this patient?

- **A.** CT scan
- **B.** IV heparin drip
- **C.** Ankle-brachial index
- **D.** Bedrest with lower extremity elevation
- **E.** Venous duplex

152. What is the most common cause of the condition shown in this patient's angiogram (Figure 152A)?

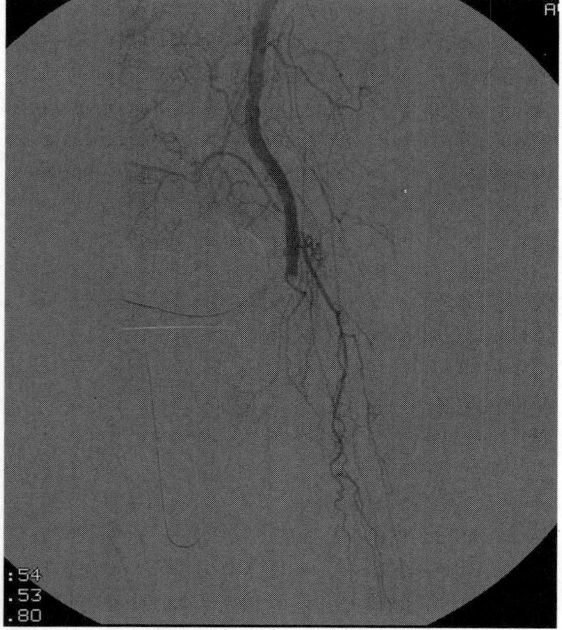

Figure 152A • Image courtesy of the University of Utah School of Medicine, Salt Lake City, Utah.

- **A.** Deep vein thrombosis
- **B.** Abdominal aortic aneurysm
- **C.** Blue toe syndrome
- **D.** Fat embolism
- **E.** Atrial fibrillation

153. What is the most appropriate treatment for this patient?

A. Systemic anticoagulation
B. Stent placed angiographically
C. Femoral artery to tibial artery bypass
D. Embolectomy
E. Medical management

End of set

---

154. You are the general surgery intern on call at a busy university hospital. You are called by the ER physician to see a 57-year-old female complaining of abdominal pain. Six months ago the patient was diagnosed with metastatic breast cancer and she has been receiving chemotherapy, with her last dose being 6 days ago. The patient states that the abdominal pain started this morning and has become progressively worse, with multiple bouts of emesis. The patient's abdomen is very tender to the touch and demonstrates rebound tenderness throughout. The patient also denies flatus or a bowel movement. A CBC reveals WBC 0.15K, HCT 20%, and Plt 65,000. A chest x-ray is obtained (Figure 154A). What is the most appropriate next step in this patient's management?

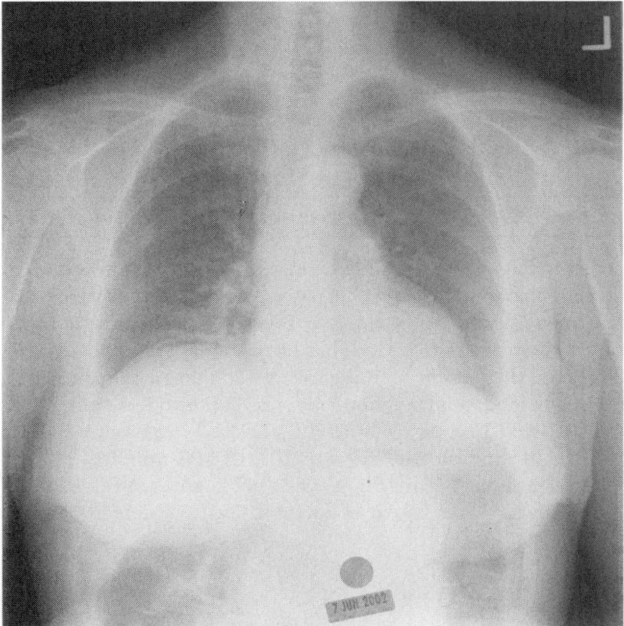

Figure 154A • Image courtesy of the University of Utah School of Medicine, Salt Lake City, Utah.

A. CT scan of the abdomen
B. Fluid resuscitation and pain control
C. Exploratory laparotomy
D. Colonoscopy
E. Plan for discharge with narcotics

155. A 12-year-old male is seen in the ED after being hit by a car. His only injury is a left closed tibia/fibula fracture. The orthopedic surgeon on call takes the patient to the operating room and performs an open reduction with internal fixation. Later that night the patient complains of increasing left leg pain, unrelieved with morphine. After the dressings are removed, a tight left lower leg is noted. The dorsal pedal pulse is palpable, but the patient is unable to move his toes and cries out in pain upon passive dorsal flexion. What is the most appropriate next step?

- **A.** Four-compartment fasciotomies
- **B.** A different narcotic
- **C.** Surgical embolectomy
- **D.** Duplex Doppler scan
- **E.** Nothing, as long as you can feel pulses

156. An 18-year-old motorcycle rider is admitted to the ER after suffering a closed head injury with loss of consciousness. The patient's vital signs are as follows: BP 128/74, HR 85, RR 18, T 38°C, and GCS 10. The patient is also confused and combative. The trauma evaluation shows no associated injuries other than a scalp laceration. After appropriate treatment you suspect post–head injury diabetes insipidus. Which of the following findings is most consistent with this diagnosis?

- **A.** High urine specific gravity
- **B.** Low urine output
- **C.** Polydipsia
- **D.** Low serum sodium
- **E.** Fluid restriction

The next two questions (items 157 and 158) correspond to the following vignette.

A 75-year-old male is transferred from a nearby skilled nursing facility to the emergency department because of increasing abdominal pain. The patient has a history of dementia and has been a resident of this facility for approximately 5 years. A nurse who accompanies him to the hospital tells you that the patient has not eaten anything for 2 days and has been vomiting. On exam, the patient is in mild distress and has a palpable right upper quadrant mass, with a distended, tender abdomen, without peritoneal signs. Vital signs are as follows: T 36.5°C, BP 115/65, HR 95, RR 12, and SaO_2 95% on room air. Labs results are as follows: Na 145 mmol/L, K 3.5 mmol/L, Cl 103 mmol/L, HCO_3 30 mmol/L, BUN 25 mg/dL, creatinine 1.1 mg/dL, glucose 115 mg/dL, WBC 10,000, HCT 45%, Plt 450,000, and lipase 33 U/L. An abdominal film is obtained (Figure 157A).

157. What is this patient's most likely diagnosis?

- **A.** Perforated duodenal ulcer
- **B.** Diverticulitis
- **C.** Pancreatitis
- **D.** Appendicitis
- **E.** Sigmoid volvulus

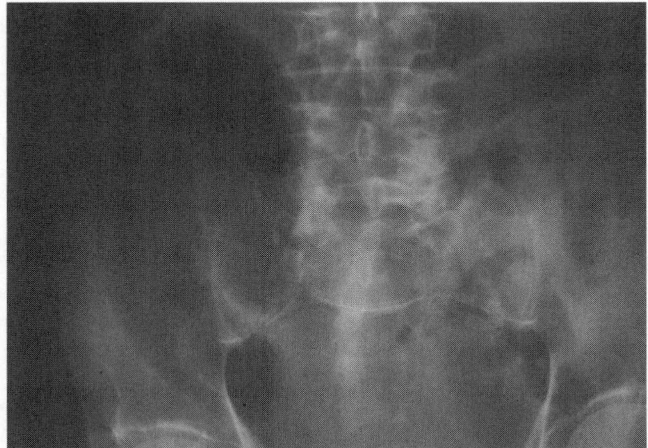

Figure 157A • Image courtesy of the University of Utah School of Medicine, Salt Lake City, Utah.

158. What is the most appropriate next step in his management?

A. Abdominal ultrasound
B. Endoscopic reduction
C. CT scan of the abdomen
D. Exploratory laparotomy
E. Observation

End of set

---

159. A 55-year-old obese female with a history of long-standing renal failure requiring dialysis is admitted to the ER with a clotted AV fistula. The patient has missed her regular dialysis and complains of fatigue, nausea, and feeling puffy. The patient's BP is 178/101, HR is 101, and RR is 22. Labs are drawn and show K 6.8 mmol/L. The patient's EKG tracing shows peaked T waves with a prolonged PR interval and widening of the QRS complex. What is the initial step in the emergency treatment of hyperkalemia?

A. Calcium gluconate
B. Metoprolol
C. Insulin and glucose
D. Dialysis
E. Albuterol

160. A 33-year-old female comes to the emergency room to be evaluated for frequent spontaneous nose bleeds. The CBC obtained reveals a WBC 9500, HCT 37%, and Plt 19,000. The patient is eventually diagnosed with ITP and given oral steroids for treatment, with follow-up appointments scheduled in oncology. Lacking health care insurance she returns to the emergency room 2 weeks after her discharge for increasing frequency and duration of nose bleeds. The patient has a platelet count of 500. What is the most appropriate next step in management of this patient?

- **A.** Outpatient follow-up only
- **B.** Prednisone, 1 mg/kg/day for 6 months
- **C.** Splenectomy
- **D.** Technetium 99-m colloid liver spleen scan
- **E.** Platelet transfusion until the count is normal

The next three questions (items 161–163) correspond to the following vignette.

A 64-year-old male presents to the emergency room with a 12-hour history of acute-onset abdominal pain. The patient states that the pain is located primarily around his umbilicus and is unremitting and intense in nature. The physical exam is concerning because pain is out of proportion to the physical findings. Past medical history is significant for diabetes mellitus and atrial fibrillation, for which the patient takes insulin and aspirin, respectively.

161. What is the most likely diagnosis?

- **A.** Gastritis
- **B.** Ruptured abdominal aortic aneurysm
- **C.** Mesenteric ischemia
- **D.** Ulcerative colitis
- **E.** Gastric tumor

162. You order a panel of labs, including a CBC, metabolic panel, hepatic panel, and an arterial blood gas. Which of the following abnormalities consistent with your diagnosis would you expect in this patient?

- **A.** Decreased hematocrit
- **B.** Metabolic acidosis
- **C.** Metabolic alkalosis
- **D.** Hyponatremia
- **E.** Decreased albumin

163. Of the following, which is the most appropriate study to obtain to confirm your diagnosis?

- **A.** Right upper quadrant ultrasound
- **B.** Colonoscopy
- **C.** Enteroclysis
- **D.** Angiogram
- **E.** Upper endoscopy

End of set

The next two questions (items 164 and 165) correspond to the following vignette.

A 33-year-old female who is 5 weeks postpartum comes to the emergency department with a 3-day history of nausea and vomiting. The patient reports normal bowel function and states that the nausea usually occurs about 1 hour after eating. On exam, the patient's abdomen is soft and nondistended, with right upper quadrant tenderness. Vital signs are as follows: BP 118/72, HR 97, and T 38.8°C. Labs are as follows: WBC 13,000, total bilirubin 1.3 mg/dL, AST 70 U/L, ALT 62 U/L, amylase 81 U/L, and lipase 110 U/L. An ultrasound of the gallbladder (Figure 164) shows gallbladder wall thickening with a small amount of pericholecystic fluid and evidence of multiple gallstones. There is no intrahepatic ductal dilation.

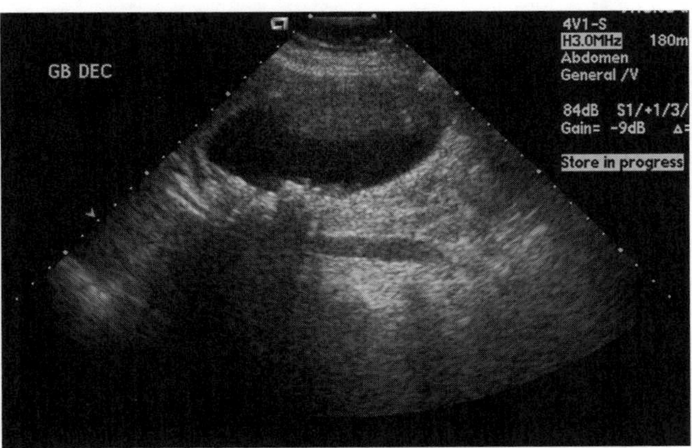

Figure 164 • Image courtesy of the University of Utah School of Medicine, Salt Lake City, Utah.

164. What is this patient's diagnosis?

- **A.** Symptomatic cholelithiasis
- **B.** Acute acalculous cholecystitis
- **C.** Acute calculus cholecystitis
- **D.** Ascending cholangitis
- **E.** Biliary dyskinesia

165. Had the ultrasound of this patient's gallbladder been normal, what study would be the next best choice to evaluate for gallbladder disease?

- **A.** Abdominal CT scan
- **B.** HIDA scan
- **C.** Oral cholecystogram
- **D.** Percutaneous transhepatic cholangiography
- **E.** ERCP

End of set

The next three questions (items 166–168) correspond to the following vignette.

A 33-year-old male construction worker comes to the emergency room with the acute onset of right groin pain after vomiting 1 hour prior to his arrival at the ER. The patient reports the pain to be constant and denies any radiation of the pain. Vital signs are as follows: BP 168/88, HR 122, and T 36.6°C. The patient's abdomen is soft and nondistended, but he has a tender, palpable mass on the right side above the scrotum. The right testicle is nontender. The patient's WBC count is 7500.

166. What is this patient's most likely diagnosis?

A. Direct inguinal hernia
B. Incarcerated inguinal hernia
C. Strangulated inguinal hernia
D. Testicular torsion
E. Hiatal hernia

167. Upon taking this patient to the operating room, what is the procedure of choice?

A. Reduction of the hernia via a groin incision
B. Exploratory laparotomy via a midline incision
C. Orchiopexy
D. Reduction in the OR under anesthesia if possible
E. Exploration and hernia repair via the groin

168. At the time of surgical repair of the hernia, you diagnose the patient with an indirect inguinal hernia based on what finding?

A. Hernia sac located anterior to the epigastric vessels
B. Hernia sac located posterior to the epigastric vessels
C. Hernia sac located medial to the inferior epigastric vessels
D. Hernia sac located lateral to the inferior epigastric vessels
E. Hernia sac protruding through Hesselbach's triangle

End of set

The next two questions (items 169 and 170) correspond to the following vignette.

A 70-year-old female comes to the emergency department 3 weeks after being discharged from the hospital for acute, uncomplicated diverticulitis that required IV antibiotic administration. Currently she complains of pain that has increased over the last 5 days. The pain is mainly in the right upper quadrant and is associated with fever, chills, and decreased appetite. Vitals signs are as follows: T 38.6°C, HR 65, BP 123/63, RR 15, and SaO_2 93% on room air. On physical exam, the patient is a slightly obese female, who has tenderness in the right upper quadrant without rebound or rigidity. A CT scan is obtained (Figure 169).

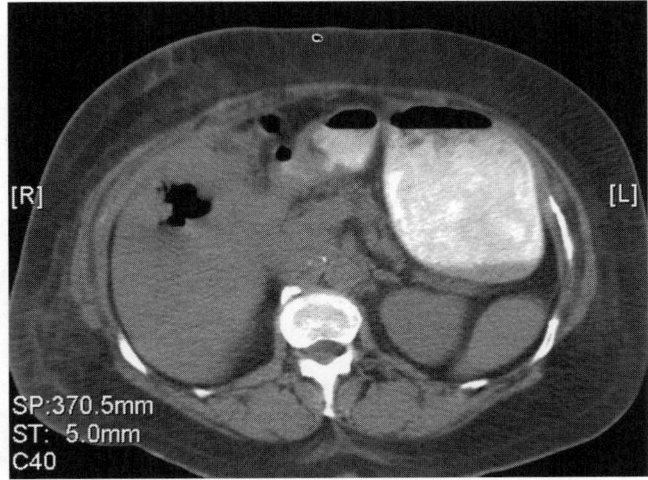

Figure 169 • Image courtesy of the University of Utah School of Medicine, Salt Lake City, Utah.

169. Which of the following conditions is the most likely cause of this patient's problem?

A. Pelvic inflammatory disease
B. Sigmoid volvulus
C. Irritable bowel syndrome
D. Diverticulitis
E. Urosepsis

170. What is the most appropriate initial therapy for this patient?

A. Broad-spectrum IV antibiotics
B. Exploratory laparotomy and hepatic resection
C. Broad-spectrum IV antibiotics with drainage via surgical laparotomy
D. Broad-spectrum IV antibiotics and percutaneous drainage
E. Oral antibiotics with follow-up in the clinic

End of set

The next two questions (items 171 and 172) correspond to the following vignette.

A 66-year-old male comes to the emergency department with the acute onset of abdominal pain that began 3 hours ago. The pain is constant and radiates to his back. Past medical history is significant for hypertension, type 2 diabetes, a significant drinking history, and a 40-pack-per-year history of smoking. The patient is anxious and diaphoretic with the following vital signs: BP 88/48, HR 122, RR 34, and T 36.2°C. You palpate his abdomen and feel a pulsatile mass.

171. What is the next step in this patient's management?

- **A.** Ultrasound of the abdomen
- **B.** CT scan of the abdomen
- **C.** Placement of 2 large-bore peripheral IVs
- **D.** Intubation
- **E.** Placement of a central line for central IV access

172. If the same patient were to present with an asymptomatic abdominal aortic aneurysm, which was found during a routine physical exam by his primary care provider, what would be the indication to repair it electively?

- **A.** Extension of the aneurysm above the renal arteries
- **B.** Extension of the aneurysm into at least one of the iliac arteries
- **C.** Diameter greater than 5 cm
- **D.** Growth in diameter greater than 3 mm annually
- **E.** Should never be electively repaired due to high operative risk

End of set

The next three questions (items 173–175) correspond to the following vignette.

A 27-year-old male is the unrestrained passenger in a car when it is broadsided at high speed. The patient is transported by air to the hospital. On arrival to the ER, he is difficult to rouse. Vitals are as follows: HR 125, BP 84/62, RR 30, and T 36.5°C. On exam, the patient has facial abrasions, decreased breath sounds on the left, a distended abdomen, and external rotation of the right femur.

173. What is the most appropriate first step in this patient's management?

- **A.** Exploratory laparotomy
- **B.** Endotracheal intubation
- **C.** Chest x-ray
- **D.** Infusion of crystalloid
- **E.** Tube thoracostomy

174. On further assessment, the patient continues to have hypotension with systolic pressures in the 80s. He is also difficult to ventilate. The chest x-ray obtained in the trauma bay is shown in Figure 174A. What action is critical in helping to stabilize this patient?

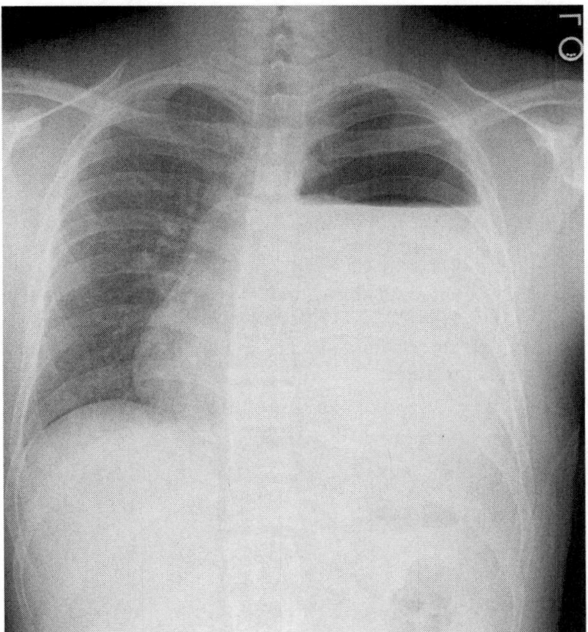

Figure 174A • Image courtesy of the University of Utah School of Medicine, Salt Lake City, Utah.

- **A.** Exploratory laparotomy
- **B.** Endotracheal intubation
- **C.** Chemical paralysis
- **D.** Infusion of crystalloid
- **E.** Tube thoracostomy

175. Despite attempts to correct this patient's hemodynamic instability, the hypotension continues. The patient has received 4 units of O-negative, packed red blood cells in addition to 4 liters of crystalloid. The blood pressure remains 82/41, with a heart rate of 123. What is the most appropriate next step in the management of this case?

- **A.** Exploratory laparotomy
- **B.** Endotracheal intubation
- **C.** CT scan of the chest
- **D.** Infusion of crystalloid
- **E.** Tube thoracostomy

End of set

176. A 28-year-old, obviously intoxicated and possibly chemically impaired, unrestrained male driver is admitted to the ER after rolling his car while attempting to evade the police. Vital signs are BP 116/62, HR 116, and RR 32. Intravenous lines were placed at the scene, and an NGT is in place. The patient is uncooperative, as well as physically and verbally abusive to the staff. Full four-point restraints are in place. The patient complains of abdominal pain, is short of breath, and randomly screams for intravenous pain medication. Which portion of this patient's management is best delayed until the secondary survey?

A. Exposure
B. Abdomen
C. Circulation
D. Disability
E. Airway

177. A 16-year-old female restrained driver is involved in a head-on collision with oncoming traffic. The patient arrives intubated to the trauma bay. After your primary assessment, the vital signs are T 36.9°C, HR 135, and BP 100/60. You obtain the chest x-ray shown in Figure 177A. Assuming the patient remains in stable condition, what study will be required to further assess for intrathoracic injury?

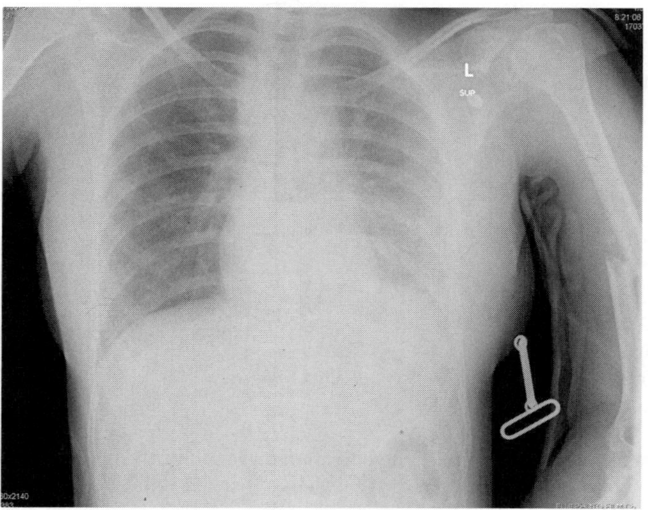

Figure 177A • Image courtesy of the University of Utah School of Medicine, Salt Lake City, Utah.

A. PA and lateral chest x-ray
B. CT of the chest
C. Thoracic arch aortogram
D. Mediastinoscopy
E. Video-assisted thoracoscopic surgery

The next two questions (items 178 and 179) correspond to the following vignette.

A 40-year-old male involved in an auto-versus-pedestrian accident arrives in the ER. The patient's vital signs are T 36.5°C, HR 140, and BP 85/40. The GCS is 15. Your exam reveals the following findings: left-sided hemotympanum with some clear discharge, multiple abrasions to the right face, the pelvis unstable to rock, and blood at the urethral meatus. On rectal exam, the tone is normal, although the prostate is difficult to palpate and gross blood is found. There is an obvious deformity to the left femur and an open fracture to the right tibia.

178. Which of the following statements is true regarding this scenario?

A. Foley catheter placement is critical in this patient to help drain the traumatized bladder.
B. Immediate head CT takes precedence over other treatments.
C. Colonoscopy should be performed to diagnose the site of bleeding.
D. The extraperitoneal bladder injury will require emergent surgery to repair it.
E. External fixation of pelvic fracture may help maintain hemodynamic stability by reducing retroperitoneal bleeding.

179. After stabilizing the patient, your further work-up reveals a transverse process fracture of the fifth cervical vertebrae. What artery must be further examined to rule out an associated injury?

A. Deep cervical artery
B. Vertebral artery
C. Ascending cervical artery
D. Common carotid artery
E. Internal carotid artery

End of set

---

180. A 77-year-old obese male with a known AAA is brought to the ER with sudden, severe abdominal pain, which radiates to his back. The patient is on diuretics for hypertension and oral medication for adult-onset diabetes. Vital signs are HR 125 and BP 88/57. The patient's abdomen is distended and mildly tender. What is the best initial management for this patient?

A. Vigorous fluid resuscitation, ICU admission for stabilization prior to operative repair
B. Paracentesis to evaluate for possible ruptured AAA
C. Emergent surgical exploration
D. Abdomen/pelvic CT scan to evaluate the AAA prior to repair
E. Emergency angiogram to confirm a ruptured AAA diagnosis

The next three questions (items 181–183) correspond to the following vignette.

A 6-year-old male is brought into the emergency room as a trauma patient after being struck by an automobile while playing in his front yard. The patient is hypotensive and has bilateral open femur fractures, from which he is hemorrhaging severely. The child is crying but his SaO_2 level is 99% on room air. You are very concerned that he will exsanguinate from his femur fractures.

181. What is the first step in the management of this patient?

- **A.** Apply direct pressure to the bleeding vessels
- **B.** Apply a tourniquet
- **C.** Transfuse type O-negative RBCs
- **D.** Obtain control of the airway
- **E.** Transfuse 2 units FFP

182. After the patient is stabilized in the trauma bay, a CT scan is obtained (Figure 182A). What injury are you concerned about after seeing this scan?

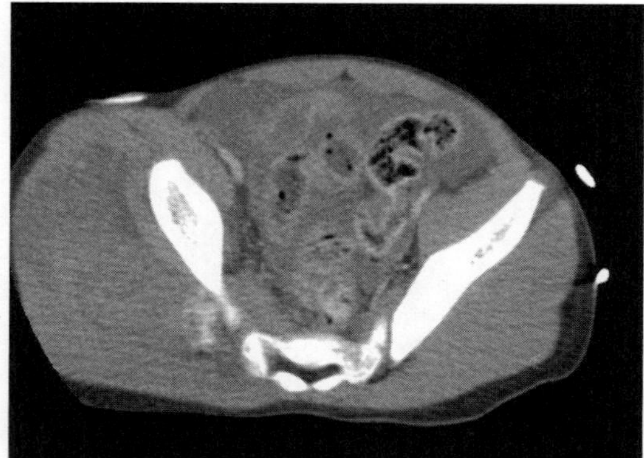

Figure 182A • Image courtesy of the University of Utah School of Medicine, Salt Lake City, Utah.

- **A.** Traumatic bowel perforation
- **B.** Splenic laceration
- **C.** Intraperitoneal bladder rupture
- **D.** Extraperitoneal bladder rupture
- **E.** Internal iliac artery injury

183. Based on your presumed diagnosis, what is the best management of this patient's condition?

- **A.** Small bowel resection
- **B.** Splenectomy
- **C.** Arterial embolization
- **D.** Suprapubic catheter placement
- **E.** Observation

End of set

The next three questions (items 184–186) correspond to the following vignette.

A 28-year-old female is ejected from her car after it is struck from the side by a car traveling approximately 50 mph. At the accident scene, her initial GCS is 10. The patient was intubated by the paramedic for respiratory distress and is brought to the emergency department in critical condition. The paramedic reports that the patient's blood pressure has been slowly falling during transport. The last pressure was 64/40 with a heart rate of 133 and an oxygen saturation rate of 62%. You notice obvious deformities of multiple ribs of the left chest.

184. What is the first step in managing this seriously injured patient?

- **A.** Administer IV fluid bolus for hypotension
- **B.** Stabilize her chest injury
- **C.** Obtain a chest x-ray
- **D.** Reevaluate the airway
- **E.** Place a central line

185. If this patient remained hypotensive and had a trachea that deviated to the right, you would be most concerned about which injury?

- **A.** Tracheal injury
- **B.** Esophageal injury
- **C.** Open pneumothorax
- **D.** Tension pneumothorax
- **E.** Flail chest

186. You determine that the patient needs a left thoracostomy tube. After placement, the chest x-ray shown in Figure 186A is obtained. What injury does this patient have?

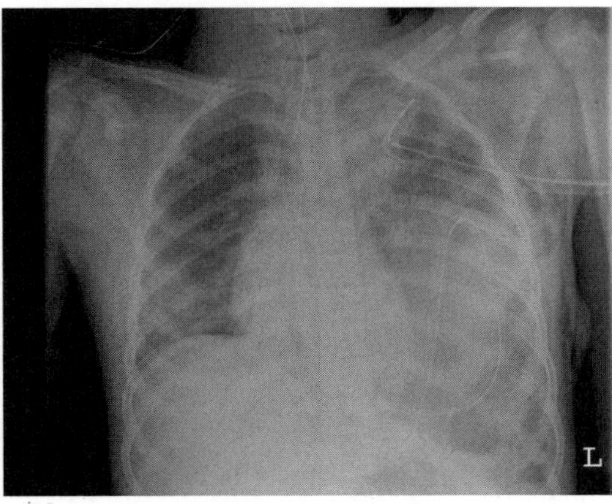

Figure 186A • Image courtesy of the University of Utah School of Medicine, Salt Lake City, Utah.

- **A.** Pulmonary laceration
- **B.** Aortic dissection
- **C.** Ruptured diaphragm
- **D.** Gastric perforation
- **E.** Cardiac contusion

End of set

187. A 32-year-old female who rolled her jeep down a nearby highway embankment is brought to the trauma bay. The patient is awake and answers questions appropriately. Primary examination shows her ABCs to be intact. The patient claims that she is unable to feel or move anything below the nipple line. Vital signs are as follows: T 37.8°C, HR 98, and BP 82/48. Fluid resuscitation is initiated. Secondary survey reveals thoracic spine tenderness and midline deformities and a large, deep abrasion to the left thigh, which is contaminated with dirt and grass. The abdomen is soft, nondistended, and nontender. An abdominal ultrasound shows no free peritoneal fluid, and laboratory values are unremarkable. One liter of crystalloid is infused without improvement in blood pressure. What is the most important medication for this patient to receive at this point?

- **A.** Cefazolin
- **B.** Methylprednisolone
- **C.** Norepinephrine
- **D.** Phenylephrine
- **E.** Morphine sulfate

The next three questions (items 188–190) correspond to the following vignette.

An 18-year-old female is seen in the ED with a 1-day history of abdominal pain. The patient states that the pain began periumbilically as a dull ache, but it has since migrated to the right lower quadrant. It is now sharp and constant in nature. This morning, the patient began vomiting and had one episode of diarrhea. She is sexually active and her last menstrual period ended 7 days ago. On exam, she is ill appearing and tachycardic. There is involuntary guarding in both quadrants of the lower abdomen. A pelvic exam reveals tenderness noted upon movement of the cervix and similar pain during rectal exam. A CBC demonstrates a leukocytosis of 13,000, and β-hCG is negative.

188. What is the most appropriate next step in the management of this patient?

- **A.** Surgical exploration
- **B.** Abdominal ultrasound
- **C.** CT scan of the abdomen
- **D.** IV hydration and observation
- **E.** Oral antibiotics and follow-up in 2 days

189. In order of decreasing frequency, what are the potential causes of appendicitis in this patient?

- **A.** Foreign body, tumor, fecalith
- **B.** Tumor, fecalith, lymphoid hyperplasia
- **C.** Fecalith, lymphoid hyperplasia, tumor
- **D.** Lymphoid hyperplasia, fecalith, tumor
- **E.** Fecalith, tumor, lymphoid hyperplasia

190. Further radiographic imaging demonstrates acute appendicitis. The patient is taken to the operating room for surgical exploration. Two days later, the pathology report reveals a 1 cm carcinoid tumor at the tip of the appendix. What further treatment should be implemented?

A. CT scan of the abdomen and pelvis for metastatic staging
B. No further treatment
C. Radiation therapy
D. Right hemicolectomy
E. Chemotherapy

End of set

The next two questions (items 191 and 192) correspond to the following vignette.

A 15-year-old female presents to the emergency department with a 2-day history of lower abdominal pain. The patient states that the pain began in the right lower quadrant, but has progressively worsened over the last 24 hours, becoming quite intense. She denies having a fever but complains of nausea, vomiting, and a poor appetite. Her last menstrual period was 6 weeks ago, and she reports being sexually active only twice. Currently she takes no medications and denies allergies. On physical exam, she appears acutely ill and has diffuse tenderness in the lower abdomen, with the right side being worse than the left, with no peritoneal signs. Rectal and pelvic exams are normal. A serum β-hCG level is 5500 mIU/mL.

191. What initial test is most appropriate in the work-up of this patient?

A. CT scan of abdomen and pelvis
B. Pelvic ultrasound
C. Abdominal series
D. Culdocentesis
E. Diagnostic laparoscopy

192. What is the most likely diagnosis?

A. Acute appendicitis
B. Acute diverticulitis
C. Ruptured ovarian cyst
D. Tubo-ovarian abscess
E. Ectopic pregnancy

End of set

The next two questions (items 193 and 194) correspond to the following vignette.

A 45-year-old male skier is brought to the emergency room by helicopter after being struck by an out-of-control snowboarder. Initially the patient was dazed and confused but these symptoms quickly resolved and he continued to ski to the lodge. The patient's wife noticed that he was acting strangely, so she took him to the clinic at the resort. From there, he was transported to the hospital. On exam, the patient has a GCS of 14, and he demonstrates some confusion, perseveration, and a slightly dilated right pupil. The patient is taken for a CT scan (Figure 193A).

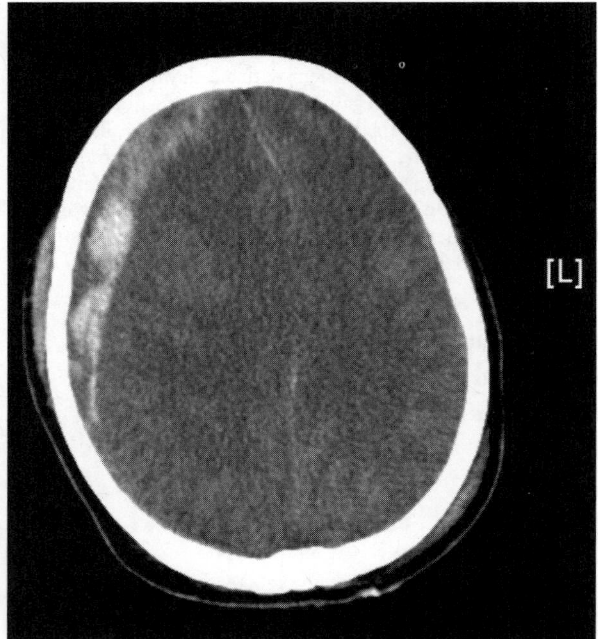

Figure 193A • Image courtesy of the University of Utah School of Medicine, Salt Lake City, Utah.

193. What is the etiology of this patient's current condition?

A. Subdural hematoma
B. Epidural hematoma
C. Subarachnoid hemorrhage
D. Intraparenchymal hemorrhage
E. Axonal shear injury

194. What is the most appropriate management option?

- **A.** Evacuation of the hematoma
- **B.** Angiographic embolization
- **C.** Ventriculostomy
- **D.** Mannitol and hyperventilation
- **E.** Serial neurological exams

End of set

The next two questions (items 195 and 196) correspond to the following vignette.

You evaluate a 42-year-old male driver in the emergency room who has been involved in a high-speed, head-on, motor vehicle accident. His GCS is 15 and after the initial ABCs of trauma care are completed, you note that the only significant injury appears to involve the patient's abdomen. The abdominal exam shows diffuse tenderness, peritoneal signs, and seat belt imprint on the lower chest and abdomen. The patient is taken to the OR; during the ensuing surgical exploration, you repair a small bowel mesentery laceration and find a large, right retroperitoneal hematoma surrounding the right kidney.

195. In what zone is this retroperitoneal hematoma found?

- **A.** Zone I
- **B.** Zone II
- **C.** Zone III
- **D.** Zone IV
- **E.** Zone V

196. What is the most appropriate management of the hematoma at this time?

- **A.** Close the abdomen and obtain a CT
- **B.** Obtain an intraoperative angiogram
- **C.** Explore the hematoma if it is expanding
- **D.** Remove the involved kidney
- **E.** Open the hematoma

End of set

The next two questions (items 197 and 198) correspond to the following vignette.

While on call in the ED, you are contacted by the medical team to see a patient with bright red blood per rectum. The patient is a 67-year-old male who was admitted 3 days ago for pneumonia. Approximately 3 hours prior to your being contacted, the patient complained of abdominal pain that was followed by passage of a large amount of stool containing gross blood. Vital signs are as follows: T 37.5°C, BP 115/76, HR 95, and SaO_2 92% on 2 L by nasal cannula. Your exam reveals an alert and responsive patient in no apparent distress. Cardiopulmonary exam reveals a regular heart rate and rhythm, skin warm and pink throughout, decreased breath sounds, and dullness to percussion in the right lower lung field. The abdominal exam is unremarkable.

197. What is the most appropriate first step in management of this patient?

A. Exploratory laparotomy
B. Endoscopy
C. Tagged RBC scan
D. CT scan
E. Angiography

198. Your initial work-up does not reveal any obvious source of bleeding but there is clearly evidence of blood in the descending colon. The patient's hematocrit remains stable and his vital signs are unchanged over the course of the next 2 days, despite ongoing bright red blood in his stool. What is the next step in this patient's management?

A. Left hemicolectomy with primary anastomosis
B. Left hemicolectomy with diverting colostomy
C. Total abdominal colectomy with ileoanal anastomosis
D. Repeat colonoscopy
E. Close observation

End of set

The next two questions (items 199 and 200) correspond to the following vignette.

A 53-year-old male presents to the emergency department after falling and striking his right lower chest. The film in Figure 199A is obtained.

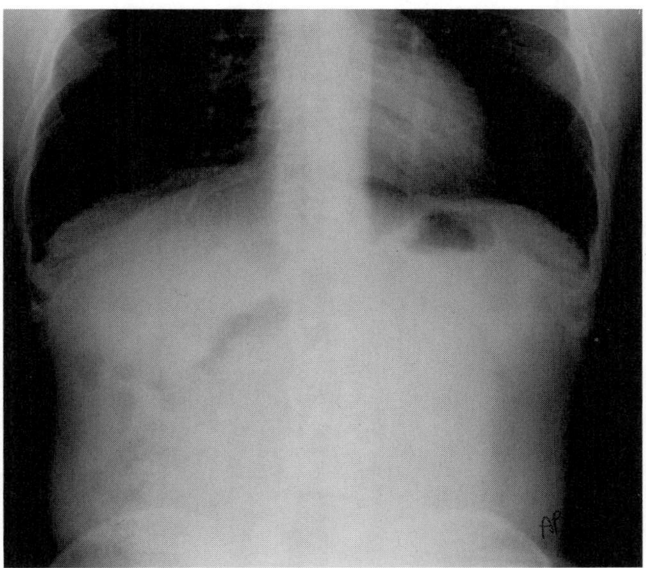

Figure 199A • Image courtesy of the University of Utah School of Medicine, Salt Lake City, Utah.

199. What is the abnormal incidental finding on the x-ray?

   A. Free intraperitoneal air
   B. Dilated small bowel
   C. A calcified gallbladder
   D. Dilated large bowel
   E. Kidney stone

200. What is the most appropriate step in this patient's management?

   A. Percutaneous transhepatic cholangiography (PTCH)
   B. Elective cholecystectomy
   C. Endoscopic retrograde cholangiopancreatography (ERCP)
   D. Emergent cholecystectomy
   E. Observation

End of set

Block

FOUR

Answers and Explanations

Block

FOUR Answer Key

151. B
152. E
153. D
154. C
155. A
156. C
157. E
158. B
159. A
160. C
161. C
162. B
163. D
164. C
165. B
166. B
167. E
168. D
169. D
170. D
171. D
172. C
173. B
174. E
175. A
176. B
177. C
178. E
179. B
180. C
181. D
182. E
183. C
184. D
185. D
186. C
187. B
188. C
189. D
190. B
191. B
192. E
193. A
194. A
195. B
196. C
197. B
198. E
199. C
200. B

151. **B.** Acute arterial occlusion is an acute event typically caused by embolization. It can also be seen in thrombosis of an atheromatous plaque or in vascular trauma. Rapid intervention is required to avoid permanent sequelae. The diagnosis is made by physical exam and is characterized by the "six P's": pain, paralysis, pallor, paresthesia, poikilothermy, and pulselessness. The most appropriate immediate treatment consists of anticoagulation with IV heparin.

A. A CT scan is an inappropriate choice for imaging because it does not evaluate peripheral arterial disease.

C. An ankle brachial index (ABI) is used to evaluate arterial insufficiency. In this patient without Doppler-able pedal signals, it will not assist in the diagnosis.

D, E. A venous duplex and bedrest with lower extremity elevation would be more appropriate in patients with venous stasis, not in patients with arterial disease.

152. **E.** An arteriogram is important to define the anatomy and demonstrate the location of vessel occlusion. The superficial femoral artery is a common site of occlusion, as shown in the angiogram in Figure 152B (note the arrow). The cause of a sudden occlusion should be determined. The most common source involves the heart; atrial fibrillation is seen in approximately 85% of all such cases. Other sources include aneurysms and atheromatous plaques proximal to the site of occlusion.

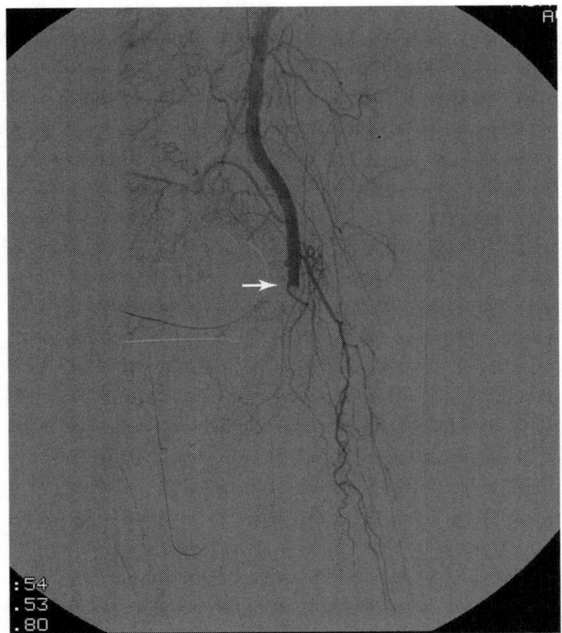

Figure 152B • Image courtesy of the University of Utah School of Medicine, Salt Lake City, Utah.

A. Deep vein thromboses are caused by venous stasis, not seen by angiography.

B. Although an abdominal aortic aneurysm can be the source of an embolism to the lower extremities, it is less likely than the most common cause, which is from the heart.

C. Blue toe syndrome occurs when atheromatous plaques are showered from the artery into the periphery. It is usually seen after cardiac catheterization.

D. A fat embolism can be seen in cases of long bone fractures. It usually occurs in the pulmonary vasculature.

153. **D.** Surgical management consists of an embolectomy, which involves cutdown of the occluded artery proximal to the occlusion with insertion of a catheter. The catheter is threaded distally until it passes the thrombus. The balloon is inflated and the catheter is withdrawn, bringing the clot along with it.

A. Anticoagulation with heparin and/or Coumadin is used as an adjunct to surgery to prevent extension or recurrence of clot formation.

B, C. Stent placement and bypass surgery are reserved for areas of atherosclerotic stenosis, not acute occlusion due to an embolism.

E. This disease is a surgical emergency, not a medically treated condition.

154. **C.** In the evaluation of an acute abdomen, the observance of pneumoperitoneum (i.e., "free air") on the chest x-ray (note the arrow in Figure 154B) or physical exam findings of peritonitis, including rebound tenderness, warrant an exploratory laparotomy. This is a surgical emergency; therefore, the other choices are inappropriate. No further radiologic evaluation is needed when a patient demonstrates peritoneal signs on physical exam and free air under the diaphragm on chest x-ray.

A. Obtaining a CT scan will delay surgical treatment and will merely show the free air already noted on the chest x-ray.

B. IV resuscitation and pain control are very appropriate, but not without an urgent laparotomy.

D. Colonoscopy would delay treatment and possibly exacerbate the problem.

E. Discharge is obviously not appropriate for a patient with an acute abdomen and free air.

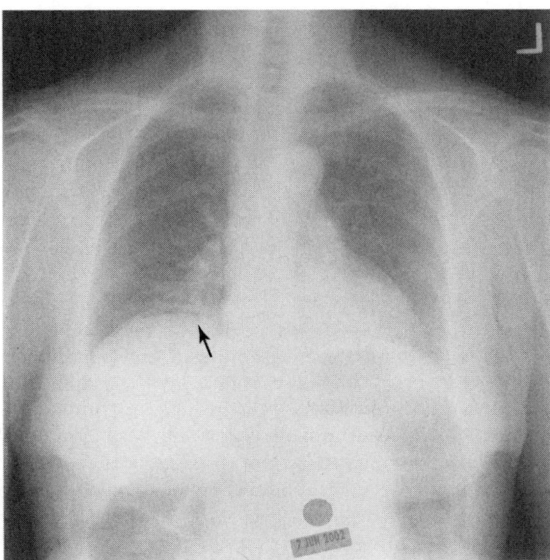

Figure 154B • Image courtesy of the University of Utah School of Medicine, Salt Lake City, Utah.

155. **A.** This case is a classic example of lower extremity compartment syndrome. Patients are at risk when reperfusion follows an extended period of ischemia. Early signs of compartment syndrome include pain out of proportion to exam, decreased sensation in the first web space, and increased pain with passive dorsiflexion of the foot. The diagnosis can be confirmed by measurement of compartment pressures; any value higher than 30 mm Hg is considered diagnostic. Patients with compartment syndrome may not lose peripheral pulses, as the pressures would have to be elevated above systolic arterial pressure to compromise arterial perfusion. Emergent four-compartment fasciotomies is the appropriate treatment.

B. Inadequate pain control is not the issue in this patient. The pain associated with compartment syndrome is significant, and trying a different narcotic will not resolve the problem.

C. There is no evidence of thrombosis formation in this case.

D. A duplex Doppler scan would show evidence of arterial flow but would miss the problem of decreased tissue perfusion.

E. Pulses may be palpable despite the presence of compartment syndrome.

156. **C.** Diabetes insipidus results from a deficiency (central DI) or unresponsiveness (nephrogenic DI) of antidiuretic hormone (ADH). Because of insensible water loss, patients experience extreme thirst.

A, B. Voluminous urine output—not low urine output—with a low specific gravity—not high specific gravity—are symptoms seen with DI.

D. Hypernatremia—not hyponatremia—is seen with DI.

E. Vasopressin and intravenous fluid replacement—not fluid restriction—are the usual means of treatment.

157. **E.** Colonic volvulus occurs when the colon twists around its mesentery, resulting in obstruction and vascular compromise. If prolonged, this condition can result in necrosis and eventually perforation. It may occur in the sigmoid colon or cecum. Sigmoid volvulus is most common, occurring in approximately 80% of cases. It is usually seen in elderly institutionalized patients with chronic constipation and history of prior abdominal surgery or distal colonic obstruction. It is characterized by acute abdominal pain, abdominal distention, and obstipation. On plain film, the "omega" sign—a loop of colon aiming toward the right upper quadrant—is commonly seen (note the arrows in Figure 157B).

A, B, C, D. Although all of these options should be part of the differential diagnosis, the history, laboratory values, and radiographic imaging help one come to the proper diagnosis.

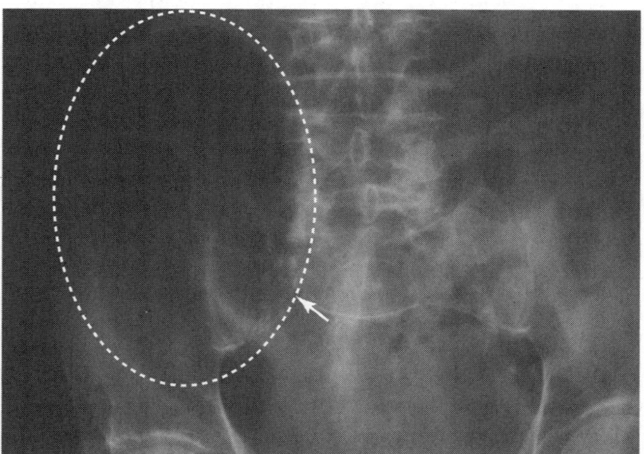

Figure 157B • Image courtesy of the University of Utah School of Medicine, Salt Lake City, Utah.

158. **B.** Sigmoidoscopy is both diagnostic and therapeutic for sigmoid volvulus and is successful in treatment of 80% of cases. Indications for surgery include free air or pneumatosis on abdominal films, peritoneal sign on exam, or unsuccessful endoscopic reduction. Most patients should undergo an elective sigmoid colectomy after reduction, as the recurrence rate for this condition approaches 40%.

A, C. Abdominal ultrasound and CT scan will help confirm the diagnosis, but they are not therapeutic.

D. The patient will require an exploratory laparotomy if the sigmoidoscopy is unsuccessful.

E. Observation is inappropriate, as continuation of this disease process will lead to bowel necrosis and perforation.

159. **A.** Hyperkalemia is seen in cases involving renal failure, crush injuries, burns, blood transfusions, iatrogenic potassium containing infusions, and secondary to some medication use. Potassium is critical to the electric physiology of the heart, and hyperkalemia can result in ventricular fibrillation and cardiac arrest. EKG findings include peaked T waves, prolongation of the PR interval, and widening of the QRS complex. Levels exceeding 6.5 mmol/L are considered critical and should be immediately addressed. Immediate treatment includes cardiac stabilization by administration of IV calcium gluconate.

B. Metoprolol is a β-antagonist and causes potassium to leave the cells and enter circulation, thereby causing hyperkalemia.

C, E. Following administration of IV calcium gluconate, you must take action to reduce the serum concentration of potassium. These steps include shifting potassium into the cells with infusion of insulin and glucose or administration of an albuterol nebulizer, diuresis of potassium with furosemide, and binding of potassium in the intestinal tract with sodium polystyrene (Kayexalate), resulting in excretion.

D. Dialysis can be used if the measures described in the explanation for C and E are ineffective or contraindicated.

160. **C.** Idiopathic thrombocytopenic purpura (ITP) is an immune condition involving antiplatelet antibodies that is most commonly seen in children younger than the age of 6 years and in women in their thirties. In children, ITP is typically self-limiting, and strict bedrest with avoidance of contact sports is recommended. The spleen is the source of the IgG specific for platelets and the site of the phagocytosis of the coated platelets. Signs and symptoms of ITP include bleeding following minor trauma, easy bruising, mucosal bleeding, and petechiae. In adults, the initial treatment includes prednisone 1 mg/kg/day, but only 25% of patients sustain their platelet levels after steroid treatment alone. In those who do not achieve a sustained response to steroid therapy, IVIG is also given. When a patient fails to respond to these medical therapies, a splenectomy is indicated. Splenectomy is successful in 85% of cases. If ITP recurs after splenectomy, it may be due to the presence of an accessory spleen. Using a technetium-99 colloid scan or infusion of indium-111–labeled platelets, accessory spleens can be localized.

A. Outpatient follow-up for a patient with severe thrombocytopenia is inappropriate and risks life-threatening complications such as spontaneous intracranial bleeding.

B. Prednisone therapy is an option but 6 months of unmonitored therapy is not indicated.

D. A radiolabeled study is used to localize splenic tissue (accessory spleens) following splenectomy. It is not indicated prior to splenectomy.

E. The spleen will continue to make antibodies to platelets, and the transfused platelets will be rapidly consumed without concurrent splenectomy.

161. **C.** Pain out of proportion to findings on physical exam is always concerning for mesenteric ischemia. Acute mesenteric ischemia can be caused by arterial thrombosis or embolus, venous occlusion, or "low flow" nonocclusive mesenteric ischemia. This patient is at higher risk for embolic disease due to his history of atrial fibrillation without adequate anticoagulation.

A. Gastritis may be painless or may be associated with less severe pain, which is typically localized in the epigastric—not periumbilical—area.

B. A patient with a ruptured abdominal aortic aneurysm is likely to be in hemorrhagic shock and have severe abdominal pain radiating to the back or groin and possibly a pulsatile abdominal mass.

D. Ulcerative colitis typically presents with crampy abdominal pain and bloody stools with a past history of the same, as well as diarrhea.

E. A gastric tumor typically presents with prolonged history of weight loss and vague upper abdominal discomfort.

162. **B.** In addition to the classic findings on a physical exam, patients with mesenteric ischemia often present with leukocytosis and metabolic acidosis (lactic acidosis). This acute condition is associated with a high mortality rate, and prompt diagnosis and treatment are imperative.

A. As a later sign of ischemic bowel, patients may develop gastrointestinal bleeding with a decrease in hematocrit, but only as a late finding, not as a presenting symptom.

C. Metabolic alkalosis may be due to over-aggressive diuresis, persistent emesis, exogenous bicarbonate loading, or a so-called contraction alkalosis. None of these findings would be expected with ischemic bowel.

D. The sodium level is not usually directly affected by ischemic bowel.

E. Decreased albumin is seen in states of chronic malnutrition, not acutely in ischemic bowel.

163. **D.** Visceral angiography is used to definitively confirm the diagnosis. Papaverine may be injected at the time of angiography to promote vasodilation.

A. Ultrasound of the right upper quadrant is used to evaluate biliary tract disease, not bowel ischemia.

B. Colonoscopy may show areas of ischemia but it is not indicated in the acute setting of bowel ischemia.

C. Enteroclysis would likely be abnormal but the test is too nonspecific and time-consuming to be helpful.

E. Upper endoscopy would likely be normal and therefore unhelpful in this acute setting.

164. **C.** This patient's condition is consistent with acute calculus cholecystitis. Cholecystitis is characterized by fever, leukocytosis, right upper quadrant tenderness, and pain. The multiple risk factors for developing gallstones include female gender, obesity, age 30 to 40 years old, and multiparity.

A. Symptomatic cholelithiasis or biliary colic causes right upper quadrant pain, usually postprandially, which may be associated with nausea and vomiting. This presentation differs from that of cholecystitis, as there is typically no fever or elevated WBC count—both indicators of inflammation.

B. Acalculous cholecystitis is not associated with gallstones. This condition is commonly seen in ICU patients or in cases where patients are NPO for acute illness.

D. Ascending cholangitis is a serious infectious process of the entire biliary tree in which bacteria (*E. coli*, *Klebsiella*, *Pseudomonas*, and *Enterococcus*) enter the bloodstream secondary to biliary obstruction. The condition is marked by fever, jaundice, and right upper quadrant pain (Charcot's triad). The addition of hypotension and mental status changes in the later stages is known as Reynolds' pentad.

E. Biliary dyskinesia is the inability of the gallbladder to empty in a normal fashion due to uncoordinated contraction of the gallbladder wall. It is not associated with a fever and elevated WBC count.

165. **B.** The test of choice to further document acute cholecystitis is a HIDA scan. In the presence of an obstructed cystic duct, intravenously administered iminodiacetic acid cannot pass into the gallbladder. The usual work-up begins with an ultrasound to document stones. When stones are not seen, a HIDA scan is the next test of choice. A normal HIDA scan shows normal filling of the gallbladder and prompt drainage into the duodenum via the common bile duct.

A. An abdominal CT scan is not helpful in documenting gallbladder function.

C. The oral cholecystogram is a test of historical interest, often unavailable today.

D. A PTHC is an invasive test to evaluate possible biliary obstruction.

E. An ERCP is an invasive procedure used to evaluate the common bile duct.

166. **B.** This patient has an incarcerated inguinal hernia. When a hernia is not able to be reduced into the abdomen, it is considered incarcerated. When blood flow is compromised, it is considered strangulated.

A. A direct inguinal hernia passes medial to the inferior epigastric vessels and through Hesselbach's triangle. This patient could have a direct hernia or indirect inguinal hernia, both of which could become incarcerated.

C. This scenario is unlikely to involve a strangulated inguinal hernia, because these patients usually present with a fever or elevated WBC count and diffuse abdominal pain. A strangulated hernia cannot be completely excluded from the list of possibilities, but is less likely, due to the short time frame of incarceration and the lack of systemic symptoms.

D. A torsed testicle is very painful, but this patient is not experiencing testicular discomfort.

E. A hiatal hernia occurs through the esophageal hiatus of the diaphragm, not seen in the groin.

167. **E.** The operation of choice is exploration with reduction and repair of the hernia. Operative options include the Marcy, Bassini, Shouldice, and McVay repairs, as well as tension-free mesh repairs such as the Lichtenstein repair. Complications to surgical repair include recurrence, hematomas, hydroceles, paresthesias, chronic pain, seromas, and testicular ischemia.

A. Reducing the hernia is part of the procedure, but repairing the defect is important to prevent recurrence.

B. A midline incision is inappropriate for a groin hernia unless compromised or dead bowel is discovered.

C. Orchiopexy is the wrong procedure, because the testicle is not involved in this case.

D. Reducing the hernia is part of the procedure, but the defect still needs to be repaired and the hernia contents inspected to ensure viability.

168. **D.** Hesselbach's triangle is formed by the inguinal ligament inferiorly, the rectus sheath medially, and the inferior epigastric vessels laterally and superiorly. A direct hernia protrudes through the triangle, medial to the epigastric vessels. An indirect hernia protrudes through the internal ring and lateral to the epigastric vessels following the path of the cord.

A, B. These are incorrect locations.

C, E. These are incorrect locations, which describe the position of a direct inguinal hernia.

169. **D.** In an older woman with a recent history of diverticulitis, the most likely etiology of such a lesion is a pyogenic (bacterial) hepatic abscess. These abscesses typically arise secondary to (1) portal vein bacteremia from diverticulitis or appendicitis, (2) biliary obstruction and cholangitis, (3) hepatic artery bacteremia from endocarditis, (4) direct extension from gangrenous cholecystitis of subhepatic abscess, (5) superinfection from a necrosing malignancy, or (6) necrosis after hepatic trauma and secondary to seeding of the hematoma.

A, E. While PID and urologic infections may present with similar symptoms, they are not associated with bacterial hepatic abscesses.

B, C. Sigmoid volvulus and irritable bowel syndrome are not associated with bacterial hepatic abscess.

170. **D.** Left untreated, a pyogenic liver abscess is uniformly fatal. Initial therapy consists of broad-spectrum IV antibiotics and CT-guided percutaneous drainage. This approach is successful approximately 80% of the time.

A. Broad-spectrum IV antibiotics alone have been used successfully in some patients, but results vary widely, and this is not the standard of care. Antibiotics alone might be used for a patient with multiple, widely distributed, small abscesses.

B. Drainage of the hepatic abscess—not hepatic resection—is needed.

C. Indications for surgical drainage would include the necessity for laparotomy for the underlying disorder, such as diverticular abscess, as well as failure to drain the abscess percutaneously.

E. Oral antibiotics with follow-up would be inadequate treatment for this seriously ill patient.

171. **D.** This patient has a pulsatile abdominal mass and is hemodynamically unstable and should be considered as having a ruptured aneurysm until proven otherwise. In this emergency situation, the first step is to obtain a secure airway. This patient should be intubated immediately.

A. An abdominal ultrasound is a good method to follow the size of an aneurysm, but it should not be used in the emergent management of an unstable patient.

B. A CT scan of the abdomen would be helpful to confirm the diagnosis of an abdominal aortic aneurysm, but obtaining it before stabilizing the patient is not appropriate.

C, E. Ideally, while you are intubating the patient, someone else is achieving IV access, either with large-bore peripheral IVs or a large central line, such as a cordis. Establishing a secure airway is the first priority.

172. **C.** Indications for elective repair of an abdominal aortic aneurysm include a diameter greater than 5 to 5.5 cm or growth in diameter of greater than 5 mm over a 1-year period.

A. While it makes the repair more difficult, extension above the renal arteries alone is not an indication to repair the aneurysm.

B. Extension into the iliac arteries is not an indication for surgery. This problem is commonly encountered and is fixed at the time of repair, but by itself it is not an indication to operate.

D. The aneurysm must grow more than 5 mm in a 1-year period to warrant elective repair.

E. This is a false statement in this scenario.

173. **B.** In all traumas, the ABCs (airway, breathing, and circulation) are the medical practitioner's first priority. In an alert patient, the airway can be assessed by asking the patient to speak and obtaining an appropriate response. In patients who are difficult to rouse, control of the airway is mandatory.

A. Although an exploratory laparotomy may eventually be necessary, the most important initial treatment is to address control of this patient's airway.

C. A chest x-ray will be required, but not before addressing the ABCs of resuscitation and trauma.

D. Infusion of crystalloid should be addressed as soon as possible, but not before a secure and patent airway is obtained.

E. A tube thoracostomy may be indicated on the right side, but securing the airway is the priority.

174. **E.** A large hemo-pneumothorax should be suspected due to the patient's continuing unstable vital signs and decreased breath sounds. This condition is easily treated in the emergency department by tube thoracostomy. An initial output of 1500 mL or 200 mL per hour for 4 hours of blood demands an emergent thoracotomy. The initial chest x-ray (see Figure 174A) shows a large hemo-pneumothorax with air fluid levels. Figure 174B shows resolution after proper placement of a tube thoracostomy.

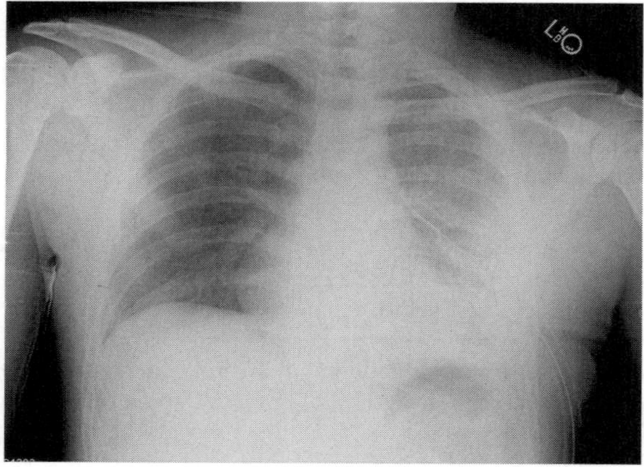

Figure 174B • Image courtesy of the University of Utah School of Medicine, Salt Lake City, Utah.

A. Currently, the most important problem this patient faces is the inability to ventilate. Taking the patient to the OR for a laparotomy is not yet indicated in this scenario.

B. The patient should already have been intubated.

C. The patient should be treated based on the physical signs. Treating the hemo-pneumothorax should improve ventilation. Chemical paralysis may merely mask an underlying situation and should be used after completing the primary and secondary trauma surveys.

D. Crystalloid infusion is a reasonable choice, but it will not correct the hemo-pneumothorax.

175. **A.** Because the airway and breathing are controlled and the patient remains in shock, the hypotension is likely due to intra-abdominal hemorrhage. The patient has not responded to an adequate trial of crystalloid infusion and blood products. To treat the patient's ongoing shock, it is imperative to take the patient to the operating room for an exploratory laparotomy.

B. The patient in this scenario should already be intubated.

C. The patient is hemodynamically unstable and should go to the operating room rather than to radiology. In situations where abdominal injury is suspected in a trauma victim with very stable vital signs, this might be the correct answer.

D. The patient has already failed infusion of 4 liters of crystalloid as well as 4 units of blood products, without improvement of vital signs.

E. A chest tube should have already been placed for the hemo-pneumothorax.

176. **B.** Abdominal evaluation for injury—in particular, for blunt injury—is part of the secondary trauma survey. The secondary survey follows the primary survey and resuscitation and involves a head-to-toe systemic assessment of the patient. It may include blood and radiologic testing as well as reassessment of the primary survey.

A. Exposure is part of the primary survey and includes completely removing all clothing and jewelry, as well as keeping the patient warm with blankets.

C. Ensuring adequate tissue circulation can be assessed through the palpation of pulses and is part of the primary survey. Once blood pressure and heart rate are assessed, resuscitation can proceed if indicated.

D. Disability is a component of the primary survey and is assessed by determining mental status, looking at the equality and reactiveness of the pupils, and performing a gross motor and sensory exam.

E. Airway is the first component of the primary survey, termed the ABCs (airway, breathing, circulation) in trauma management.

177. **C.** The chest x-ray demonstrated several nonspecific findings suggestive of an aortic injury, including widened mediastinum, apical pleural capping, loss of aortic knob, and depression of left main stem bronchus (note the arrows in Figure 177B). Traumatic aortic disruption is a highly morbid injury, with more than 85% of patients dying at the scene of the accident. In addition, there is a 50% in-hospital mortality rate for every 24 hours this injury goes undiagnosed. For these reasons, it is absolutely critical to have a high index of suspicion in trauma patients. The gold standard for diagnosing aortic injury remains angiography. The injury usually occurs just proximal to the left subclavian take-off. Treatment consists of surgical placement of an aortic interposition graft. (Note the arrows in Figures 177C and 177D.) Transesophageal echocardiogram (TEE) is rapidly becoming a useful adjunct in the rapid diagnosis of this type of injury. Because it is relatively noninvasive, it should be considered in blunt chest trauma cases. Intensive care practitioners, anesthesiologists, and cardiologists are the most likely disciplines to be trained in the use of this diagnostic method.

A. A plain film would give only the nonspecific findings mentioned in the explanation for C.

B. A routine chest CT scan is not specific enough to define this injury, although the CT angiogram is gaining acceptance for screening this injury (note the arrow in Figure 177E). Nevertheless, the aortogram remains the gold standard for diagnosis.

D. A mediastinoscopy is not indicated for assessing an intrathoracic injury, even in a stable trauma patient.

E. Video-assisted thoracoscopic surgery is not indicated in a trauma patient to evaluate a possible aortic disruption.

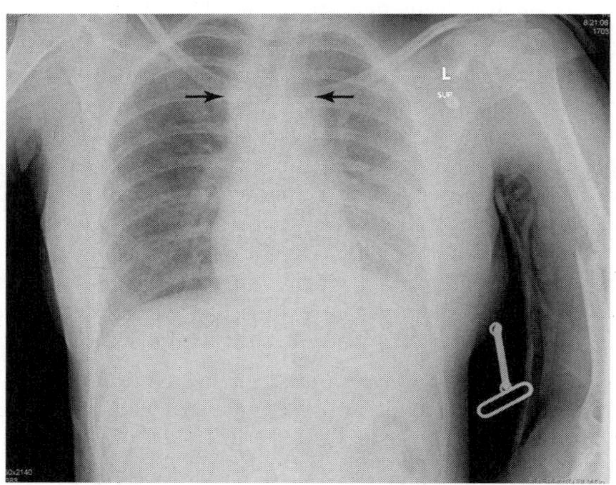

Figure 177B • Image courtesy of the University of Utah School of Medicine, Salt Lake City, Utah.

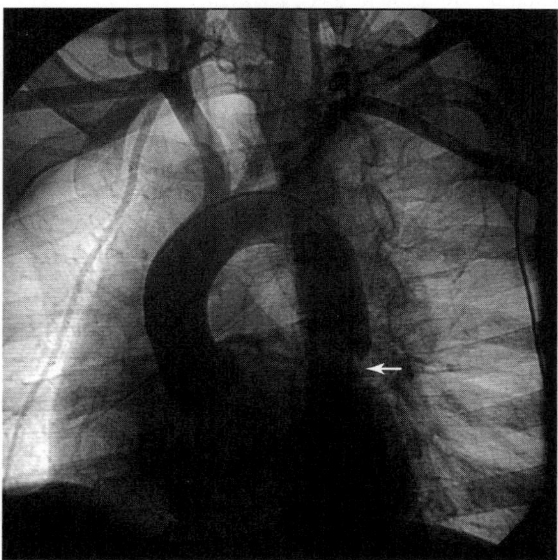

Figure 177C • Image courtesy of the University of Utah School of Medicine, Salt Lake City, Utah.

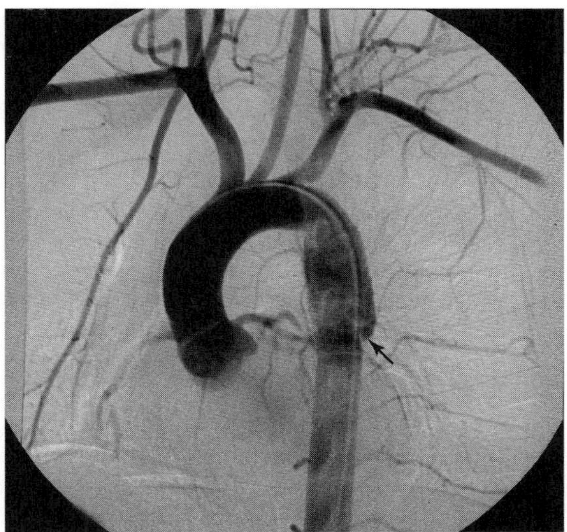

Figure 177D • Image courtesy of the University of Utah School of Medicine, Salt Lake City, Utah.

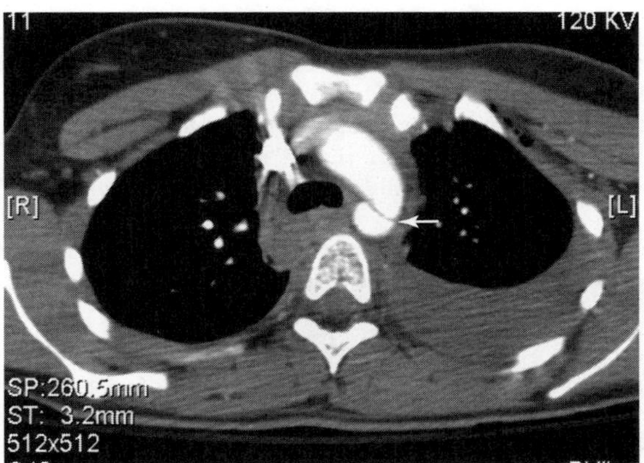

Figure 177E • Image courtesy of the University of Utah School of Medicine, Salt Lake City, Utah.

178. **E.** An open book fracture of the pelvis is common in trauma and is associated with disruption of the vertebral venous plexus along the sacrum. This type of fracture can lead to a large amount of retroperitoneal bleeding, requiring blood transfusions and aggressive resuscitation. In this orthopedic emergency, the patient should be stabilized as soon as possible to prevent massive blood loss and third spacing. A temporary method to accomplish this goal is application of MAST trousers until arrival at the trauma center. Once the patient is at the hospital, an external fixation device should be placed to reduce the fracture and help minimize retroperitoneal bleeding.

A. This patient has blood found at the external meatus, which is an indication of urethral injury. A retrograde urethrogram should be obtained prior to placement of a Foley catheter.

B. Following the ABCs of trauma is of utmost priority, and this care should be delivered first before obtaining any imaging modality.

C. Rectal injuries can occur with traumatic pelvic fractures. Proctoscopy or flexible sigmoidoscopy can be used to help diagnose the location of the lesion, although this is not the most urgent treatment option at this time.

D. Extraperitoneal injuries to the bladder are associated with pelvic fractures, especially when the superior and inferior pubic rami are involved. This type of injury is treated nonsurgically with placement of a Foley catheter for a prolonged period of time.

179. **B.** The vertebral artery courses through the transverse foramina of the second through sixth cervical vertebrae. Any fracture through the transverse foramen at this level may cause a disruption or dissection of the vertebral artery. This type of fracture warrants a CT angiogram or invasive angiogram of the vertebral artery to verify patency.

A, C, D, E. The deep cervical, ascending cervical, common carotid, and internal carotid arteries do not flow through the cervical transverse foramina.

180. **C.** Survival after ruptured AAA is dependent on rapid diagnosis and immediate surgical exploration for repair. A ruptured AAA carries a 90% overall mortality rate, which can be reduced to 50% for patients who reach a hospital that is capable of providing appropriate care via immediate exploration and repair. Figure 180 is an abdominal CT showing a rim of calcium at the borders of the AAA and surrounding retroperitoneal hematoma from rupture (note the arrow).

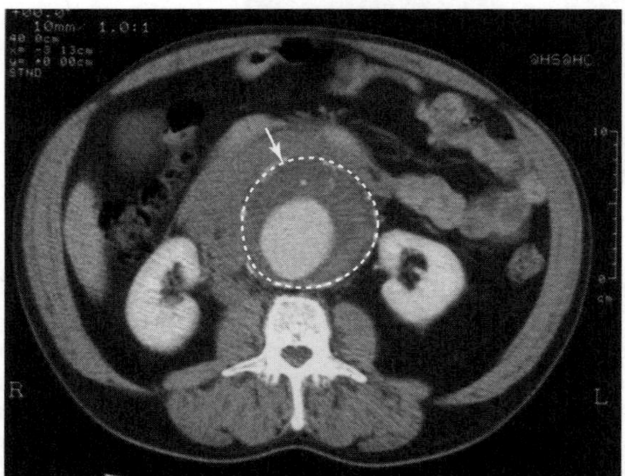

Figure 180 • Image courtesy of the University of Utah School of Medicine, Salt Lake City, Utah.

A. While fluid resuscitation for hypovolemic shock is needed, once the diagnosis of AAA rupture is made, surgical exploration and repair should not be delayed for attempts at stabilization.

B. An acute AAA rupture, as described in this case, usually consists of a rupture with the surrounding hematoma contained within the retroperitoneum. Paracentesis in an effort to find evidence of rupture would therefore be fruitless and needlessly delay the proper surgical treatment.

D. The CT scan is an excellent diagnostic tool for evaluating patients suspected of having an AAA. However, in the setting of suspected ruptured AAA, obtaining a CT scan would merely delay the move to immediate surgical care.

E. While abdominal angiography is a test for work-up of some aortic aneurysms, it should not be used to confirm a ruptured AAA. Time wasted in obtaining the study could potentially be lethal due to delay in definitive surgical care.

181. **D.** This critically ill young boy may be bleeding to death from his numerous injuries. Despite the severity of his injuries and the fact that he appears to be oxygenating well, the first step is to establish a secure airway. In a trauma situation, airway, breathing, and circulation take priority, and should be addressed in that order. Controlling the bleeding and giving red blood cells (RBCs) and fresh frozen plasma (FFP) are secondary to obtaining a secure airway.

A, C, E. Applying pressure to bleeding vessels and fluid resuscitation are important measures and need to be performed expediently, but only after the airway is secure.

B. A tourniquet is not used in the trauma situation. Direct pressure to the bleeding vessels is required.

182. **E.** Figure 182B is a single image of the pelvis that shows a thickened bowel wall, consistent with prolonged hypotension, as well as a large gluteal hematoma. Adjacent to the hematoma is a blush indicating ongoing bleeding, which would be consistent with an arterial injury.

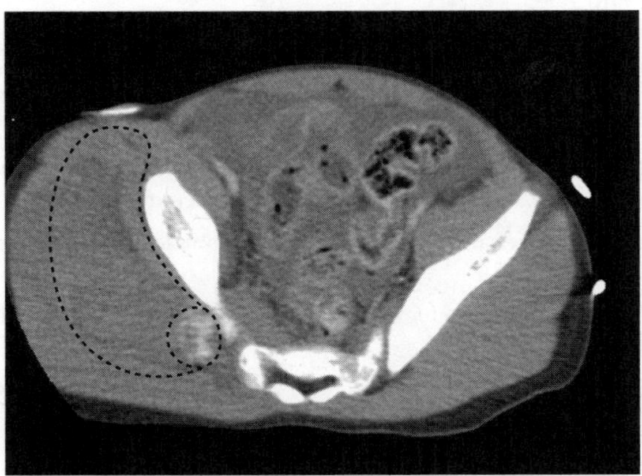

Figure 182B • Image courtesy of the University of Utah School of Medicine, Salt Lake City, Utah.

A. There is no evidence of free air indicating bowel perforation. Often in a trauma situation, bowel perforations are late findings that present 12 to 24 hours after the injury.

B. The spleen is not seen, and a diagnosis of splenic laceration cannot be made based on this scan.

C, D. There is no evidence of either intraperitoneal or extraperitoneal bladder rupture on this film.

183. **C.** With ongoing bleeding from an arterial source in a patient who is hypotensive, arterial embolization is indicated. Pelvic bleeding is difficult to control operatively; thus angiography is a valuable option. Patients may bleed from fractures, the sacral venous plexus, the major venous vessels, or arterial sources. Venous bleeding can often be controlled with external fixation, while embolization is a better option with arterial bleeds.

A. A bowel resection would not be indicated as this patient has not suffered a bowel injury.

B. A splenectomy is not indicated, as no splenic injury is seen (see Figure 181B).

D. Suprapubic catheter placement is not an option, as no bladder injury or rupture is noted.

E. Observation of a hemodynamically unstable patient is never a correct answer.

184. **D.** This critically ill patient is in shock and has obvious serious injuries. In any trauma situation, one always begins with the basics: airway, breathing, and circulation. Because this patient is critically injured, it is vital to secure the airway. Despite the fact that she is already intubated, it is important to confirm the placement of the endotracheal tube, which is evident by the poor oxygen saturation level. Often it is easier to reintubate the patient to guarantee that the endotracheal tube is in the correct position. This measure should be taken before moving to the next step.

A. While this patient's hypotension is very concerning and needs to be promptly addressed, you still start by securing the airway before addressing the other issues. Often, these tasks are being accomplished simultaneously; if not, always follow the ABCs.

B. If tension pneumothorax is suspected, a needle thoracostomy may be indicated. The first step, however, is always to make sure the airway is secure.

C. A chest x-ray is important to evaluate for chest injuries but securing the airway takes precedence.

E. Placing a central line falls under circulation, which is secondary to establishing an airway.

185. **D.** In a patient who is hypotensive, is hypoxic, and has tracheal deviation, tension pneumothorax is the diagnosis until proven otherwise. This life-threatening condition must be addressed immediately. If a tube thoracostomy is not immediately available, you might start by needling the chest to relieve the tension pneumothorax, followed by placement of a chest tube.

A, B. Tracheal and esophageal injuries are much less common in the acute, blunt trauma setting. Nevertheless, they should be kept in mind during the trauma work-up.

C. An open pneumothorax is a life-threatening injury but it does not cause tracheal deviation.

E. Flail chest occurs when a segment of chest wall does not have continuity with the rest of the thoracic cage, due to multiple rib fractures. A free-floating segment of ribs moves inward on inspiration, while the rest of the chest moves outward, referred to as paradoxical respiration. Tracheal deviation is not a usual sign of this type of injury.

186. **C.** The chest x-ray (see Figure 186A) clearly demonstrates a nasogastric tube that is in the stomach and located above the normal level of the diaphragm. This finding is consistent with a diaphragmatic rupture. Figure 186B is a CT scan that shows the stomach in the left chest, which is also consistent with a diaphragmatic rupture. Diaphragmatic rupture is a severe injury, and one that is seen most often with blunt trauma. The diagnosis is usually and easily made with a chest x-ray, with the bowel seen within the chest. The left hemidiaphragm is injured more often, as the liver is thought to offer some protection to the right hemidiaphragm.

A. Pulmonary laceration is difficult to diagnose via chest x-ray alone. It would present with lung density due to parenchymal bleeding.

B. Aortic dissection would show a widened mediastinum on chest x-ray in a hemodynamically labile patient.

D. A gastric perforation should show free air on chest x-ray.

E. A cardiac contusion would not be seen on chest x-ray.

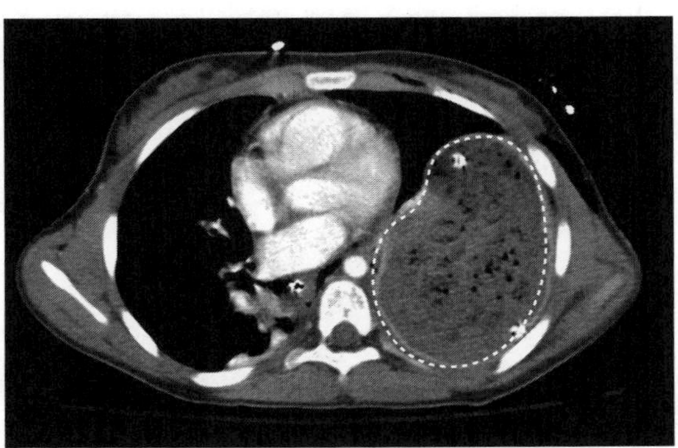

Figure 186B • Image courtesy of the University of Utah School of Medicine, Salt Lake City, Utah.

187. **B.** Injury or disruption of the spinal cord at the cervical or high thoracic level can result in the loss of autonomic innervation. The severity of complications from spinal cord injury can be significantly decreased by limiting the swelling around the cord. Steroids are known to improve the outcome if they are given within 8 hours of injury. There is no proven benefit to giving steroids after that time frame.

A. Cefazolin is a first-generation cephalosporin that provides good antibiotic coverage for skin flora. Although the patient should receive an appropriate antibiotic, it is not the most important medication at this time.

C, D. This patient is hypotensive due to decreased vascular tone from the spinal cord injury. Initially, the patient needs fluids to help maintain blood pressure. Vasoactive agents are not needed at this time.

E. Morphine sulfate is a narcotic that is commonly prescribed for trauma patients. This patient is not having any sensation due to the spinal cord injury and is not in need of pain medication. She is also hypotensive, and narcotics typically decrease blood pressure, which at this point may further complicate the picture.

188. **C.** The CT scan is becoming an important tool in diagnosing acute appendicitis, especially in young females and in patients with atypical symptoms. This patient is a good candidate for CT scan because the management of her case would likely change depending on the radiographic findings. Finding an appendix with a diameter greater than 6 mm, with thickened walls and periappendiceal fat stranding, is diagnostic for appendicitis.

A. This patient has a history and exam that are consistent with acute appendicitis. However, women of reproductive age pose a diagnostic dilemma when it comes to lower abdominal pain. Ectopic pregnancy, ovarian torsion, pelvic inflammatory disease, tubo-ovarian abscess, and ruptured ovarian cysts should all be included in the differential diagnosis. A CT scan of the abdomen would be the next step in this scenario rather than surgical exploration.

B. Abdominal ultrasound is especially helpful to diagnose lower abdominal pain in women of reproductive age, looking for ovarian pathology. Ultrasound is user dependent and not as reliable as a CT scan.

D. Although IV hydration is required, the appendicitis will not get better with fluids alone. Instead, this condition requires an operation before perforation of the appendix occurs. Observation is not an appropriate choice in this scenario.

E. Acute appendicitis is a surgical emergency, for which giving oral antibiotics with a 2-day follow-up is entirely inappropriate.

189. **D.** All of the choices listed are all causes of appendiceal lumen obstruction that cause appendicitis, with the proper order of incidence being lymphoid hyperplasia, fecalith, and tumor. Sixty percent of cases are caused by lymphoid hyperplasia, with peak incidence occurring in the teenage years. The hyperplasia leads to venous obstruction, followed by arterial insufficiency and ischemic necrosis of the appendix, which causes the pain to become localized to the right lower quadrant. Fecaliths are identified in 20% to 30% of appendicitis cases and are more commonly seen in adults. They can sometimes be identified in the right lower quadrant on abdominal plain films or on CT scans, and they need to be removed with the appendix at the time of surgery. The most common appendiceal tumor is a carcinoid. These uncommon tumors are usually located in the tip of the appendix and are unlikely to cause acute appendicitis.

A. Foreign bodies, such as seeds, can result in luminal obstruction leading to appendicitis. This is rare, however.

B, C, E. These options are all causes of appendiceal lumen obstruction, but are not arranged in the correct order of frequency.

190. **B.** The most common tumor of the appendix is a carcinoid tumor. Benign tumors, including carcinoids, are found in fewer than 5% of appendix specimens examined microscopically. They are most commonly found incidentally at the time of an appendectomy being performed for acute appendicitis. Tumors smaller than 2 cm in the tip of the appendix are unlikely to metastasize. Most authors recommend appendectomy for tumors less than 2 cm. Appendectomy alone is adequate treatment unless lymph nodes are visibly involved, the tumor is larger than 2 cm in diameter, mucinous elements are present in the tumor (adenocarcinoid), or the mesoappendix or base of the cecum is invaded.

A. No staging is required due to the low probability of metastatic disease.

C, E. Radiation therapy and chemotherapy have no role in the treatment of localized carcinoid tumors.

D. For tumors larger than 2 cm or with more aggressive lesions, the patient should undergo a right hemicolectomy.

191. **B.** A pelvic ultrasound is a safe, accurate, and useful technique in pregnant patients suspected of having an ectopic pregnancy. This procedure can identify an intrauterine pregnancy with considerable accuracy, effectively ruling out ectopic pregnancy. It should be the first imaging study performed.

A. Although a CT scan may ultimately be needed, it is not the test of choice in a female with an early pregnancy because of the risks associated with radiation exposure.

C. An abdominal series is a nonspecific test that would not be helpful in ruling out an ectopic pregnancy and would expose an early pregnancy to unnecessary radiation.

D. Culdocentesis is a diagnostic procedure that was more commonly used prior to the routine use of ultrasonography. It entails placing an 18-gauge needle in the cul-de-sac of Douglas and aspirating the contents. A negative culdocentesis cannot definitively confirm or rule out an ectopic pregnancy.

E. A diagnostic laparoscopy is a reasonable option, but only in cases in which other noninvasive modalities are unable to confirm a diagnosis.

192. **E.** Ectopic pregnancy should be high on the differential diagnosis of a woman of reproductive age with abdominal pain. Its incidence has increased over the past few years secondary to an increase in the incidence of pelvic inflammatory disease (PID). An ectopic pregnancy usually occurs after implantation of the embryo in the fallopian tube; this tube is not suited to accommodating the conceptus. The growing conceptus will eventually erode into blood vessels or cause the fallopian tube to rupture. Delay in diagnosis can lead to catastrophic bleeding and maternal death. Patients usually present with abdominal pain, amenorrhea, and vaginal bleeding. The diagnosis is made by obtaining a β-hCG level and a pelvic ultrasound. Traditional treatment has consisted of surgical removal, although some ectopic gestations may be treated with methotrexate.

A. Acute appendicitis should always be on the differential diagnosis list at this point. The clinical presentation in this case and the positive pregnancy test warrant investigation of an ectopic pregnancy. In cases of appendicitis pelvic ultrasound may reveal a noncompressible, fluid-filled tubular structure in the right lower quadrant with a diameter greater than 6 mm.

B. Acute diverticulitis is more common in older patients. It would be extremely unlikely in such a young female.

C. A ruptured ovarian cyst should be high on the differential diagnosis list in a woman of reproductive age. A CT scan can be helpful for distinguishing the etiology of the pain. A ruptured cyst would most likely demonstrate free pelvic fluid without an adnexal mass.

D. Tubo-ovarian abscesses develop in approximately 15% of women with PID and can often mimic appendicitis. Risk factors for developing PID include multiple sexual partners, previous PID, and use of an intrauterine device for birth control. Treatment of an abscess would include surgical drainage and IV antibiotics. Complications of infertility may occur from severe scarring caused by PID, and affected women have an increased risk for ectopic pregnancy.

193. **A.** Transection of the cerebral veins as they enter the superior sagittal sinus is the most common cause of a traumatic subdural hematoma. Blood collects below the dura and above the subarachnoid membranes. Initially, the bleeding is not enough to cause noticeable symptoms. As the hematoma increases in size, however, the underlying brain becomes compressed, causing symptoms of increased intracranial pressure. The CT in Figure 193B (note the arrows) shows a concave-shaped hematoma on the right, which is displacing the brain to the left.

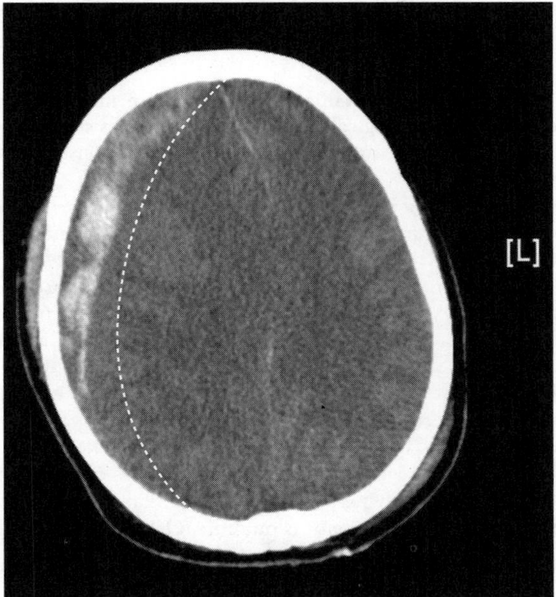

Figure 193B • Image courtesy of the University of Utah School of Medicine, Salt Lake City, Utah.

B. Epidural hematomas are usually the result of blunt trauma to the head leading to arterial bleeding from the middle meningeal artery. They are often associated with temporal skull fractures. The patient typically experiences a brief loss of consciousness, which is followed by several hours of lucid behavior, and then by a rapid decline in consciousness. Diagnosis is made by CT scan of the head, demonstrating a convex-shaped hematoma with or without mass effect.

C. A subarachnoid hemorrhage usually occurs due to rupture of a cerebral aneurysm.

D. Intraparenchymal hemorrhage presents with blood within the brain parenchyma. The CT scan shown here is not consistent with an intraparenchymal bleed.

E. Axonal shear injury occurs with angular acceleration–deceleration injuries. Shearing of deep white matter tracts leaves the patient with a very low GCS and poor prognostic outcome. An MRI is the most useful radiographic modality to delineate areas of shear injury.

194. **A.** Although the majority of patients with a small subdural hematoma can be observed, any alteration in consciousness or the neurological function of the patient requires emergent surgical evacuation of the hematoma.

B. Angiographic embolization will not fix the mass effect of the hematoma, and embolizing the cerebral vessels is very unlikely.

C. Ventriculostomy is performed to monitor intracranial pressures. It is not a therapeutic maneuver.

D. IV mannitol administration and hyperventilation are used to help reduce intracranial pressure. These measures can be initiated, but definitive treatment consists of evacuation of the hematoma.

E. Observation, with serial neurologic exams, is appropriate in individuals with small hematomas and minimal neurological deficits. These patients should be observed in a critical care setting with frequent neurological examinations and immediate access to drainage if required.

195. **B.** In evaluation of abdominal trauma, the retroperitoneum is divided into three zones. Zone I (the central zone) contains the majority of the vasculature within the abdomen (i.e., the aorta, vena cava, celiac trunk, and mesenteric arteries). This zone should always be explored in both penetrating and blunt trauma. Zone II (the lateral zone) lies on either side of Zone I. The kidneys and their vasculature are found within this area. Exploration should be undertaken in penetrating trauma, or in blunt trauma with a pulsatile expanding hematoma. Zone III consists of the pelvic retroperitoneum; the iliac vessels and the hypogastric plexus are found here. This is a difficult area to explore, and obtaining hemostatic control is challenging. Mandatory exploration should occur in penetrating trauma cases. In cases involving blunt trauma, exploration should be undertaken if the hematoma is expanding or is pulsatile. Otherwise, no exploration is the best management choice.

A, C. See the explanation for B.

D, E. There are only three zones of the retroperitoneum.

196. **C.** Exploration of the hematoma—but only if it is expanding or is very large—is the correct choice. Although most lateral retroperitoneal hematomas are small and nonexpanding and do not require exploration, large, expanding, or pulsatile hematomas around the kidney require this step to control bleeding.

A. To close the abdomen and obtain a CT scan are reasonable options if the hematoma is small and not expanding.

B. It would be technically difficult, if not impossible, to obtain an intraoperative angiogram that accesses the renal blood flow and offers the detail needed to evaluate a renal vascular injury.

D. Removing the involved kidney may be needed for major vascular injuries. In the majority of cases, blunt renal trauma is contained by Gerota's fascia. When this condition is conservatively treated with observation, patients have a reasonable rate of healing with normal renal function.

E. Opening the hematoma regardless of size or position is incorrect. Lateral retroperitoneal injuries (Zone II) and pelvic hematomas (Zone III) do not routinely require exploration, unlike upper central retroperitoneal hematomas (Zone I), which should be explored because of the high rate of associated vascular and pancreatic injuries.

197. **B.** Acute lower gastrointestinal (GI) hemorrhage is defined as continuous bleeding from the rectum, with or without hemodynamic instability. Aggressive fluid resuscitation should be initiated in an ICU setting during work-up of the etiology. A nasogastric tube should be inserted and aspirated to eliminate the possibility of a massive upper GI bleed. Endoscopy, including colonoscopy and esophagogastroduodenoscopy, is a critical step in the management of a lower GI bleed. Cauterization can be therapeutic if the site of active bleeding is identified. Colonoscopy is successful in localizing the bleeding site(s) in 50% to 90% of cases, according to clinical trials.

A. Exploratory laparotomy may be required in an unstable patient or after unsuccessful endoscopy. If the source of bleeding is not localized, a total colectomy may be the only option.

C. Tagged RBC scans may be obtained to localize the bleeding following a negative endoscopy in a stable patient. Unfortunately, localization with this procedure is not entirely dependable. If the scan is positive, the patient should proceed to angiography for further delineation and treatment.

D. A CT scan would yield little information in an acute intestinal bleeding scenario.

E. Angiography may be used to localize the bleeding vessel and treat it with embolization. This technique is best employed following localization with a tagged RBC scan.

198. **E.** Given that the patient is not currently experiencing any hemodynamic compromise and does not require transfusions for his hematocrit, there is no urgency for surgery. Approximately 80% to 90% of lower GI bleeds will stop spontaneously, making close observation the appropriate next step.

A, B, C. Given that the patient is hemodynamically stable and does not require transfusions, there is no need for urgent surgery.

D. Repeating the colonoscopy at this time is not necessary, as the patient is clinically doing well. If the bleeding became more brisk and intervention became necessary, repeating the colonoscopy would be the next logical step.

199. **C.** Figure 199B shows a calcified gallbladder (see the arrow). Also known as a porcelain gallbladder, it is usually discovered incidentally radiographically, on physical exam, or during surgery for another condition. It is thought to develop secondary to recurrent inflammation from gallstones, although most patients remain asymptomatic.

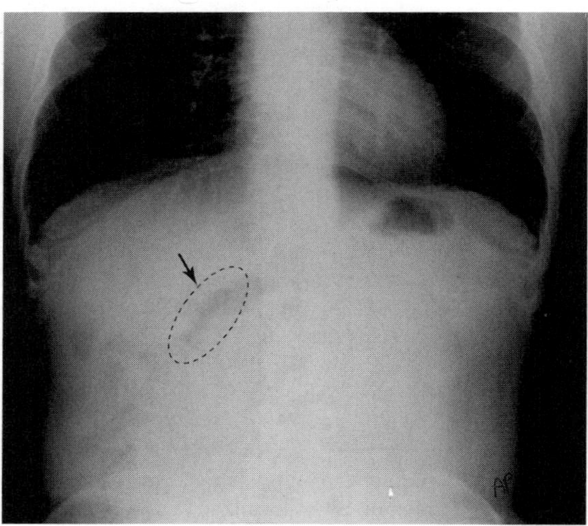

Figure 199B • Image courtesy of the University of Utah School of Medicine, Salt Lake City, Utah.

A. Free intraperitoneal air below the diaphragm would be evident on an upright film. In patients who are unable to be upright, a left lateral decubitus can be obtained, where free air will be seen overlying the liver. This patient does not have any free air on this film.

B, D. The bowel gas patterns are normal on this film.

E. Approximately 80% of all renal stones are visible on abdominal plain films, but they are not seen here.

200. **B.** Elective cholecystectomy is the treatment of choice, as there may be an increased incidence of gallbladder carcinoma in patients with a porcelain gallbladder.

A. A PTCH would be used to evaluate or drain the biliary tree, but it is not indicated here.

C. An ERCP would be used to evaluate the biliary and pancreatic ductal systems, but it is not indicated here.

D. Although cholecystectomy is strongly recommended, it can be done as an elective procedure as there is no indication for emergency surgery.

E. Observation is not recommended due to the risk of gallbladder cancer.

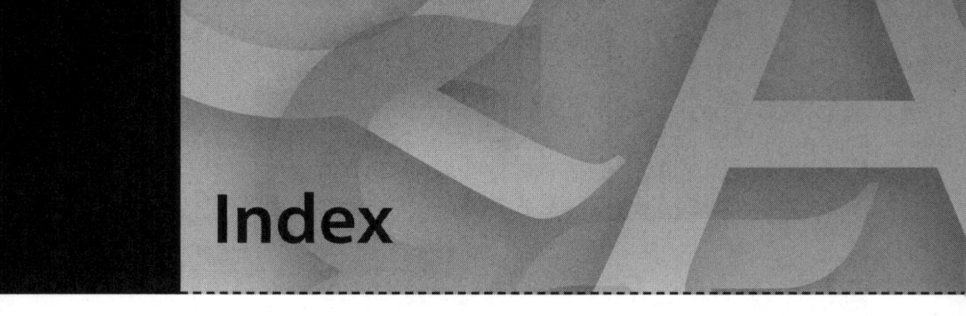

*Index note: page references with an f or a t indicate a figure or table on designated page; page references in **bold** indicate discussion of the subject in the Answers and Explanations sections.*